Breathe & Bloom 2

**Copyright © Redom Books 2025
All rights reserved.**

The content contained within this book may not be reproduced, duplicated or transmitted without direct written permission from the author or the publisher.

Under no circumstances will any blame or legal responsibility be held against the publisher, or author, for any damages, reparation, or monetary loss due to the information contained within this book. Either directly or indirectly. You are responsible for your own choices, actions, and results.

Legal Notice:

This book is copyright protected. This book is only for personal use. You cannot amend, distribute, sell, use, quote or paraphrase any part, or the content within this book, without the consent of the author or publisher.

Disclaimer Notice:

Please note the information contained within this document is for educational and entertainment purposes only. All effort has been executed to present accurate, up to date, and reliable, complete information. No warranties of any kind are declared or implied. Readers acknowledge that the author is not engaging in the rendering of legal, financial, medical or professional advice. The content within this book has been derived from various sources. Please consult a licensed professional before attempting any techniques outlined in this book.

By reading this document, the reader agrees that under no circumstances is the author responsible for any losses, direct or indirect, which are incurred as a result of the use of the information contained within this document, including, but not limited to, — errors, omissions, or inaccuracies.

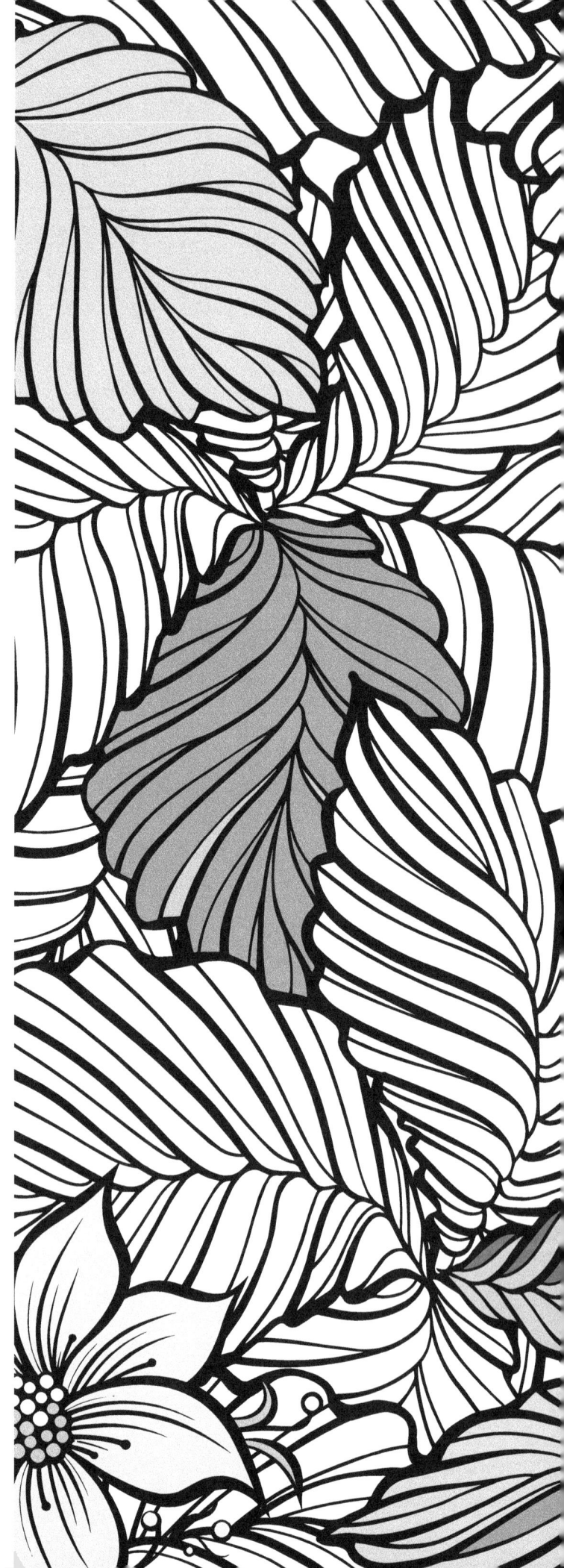

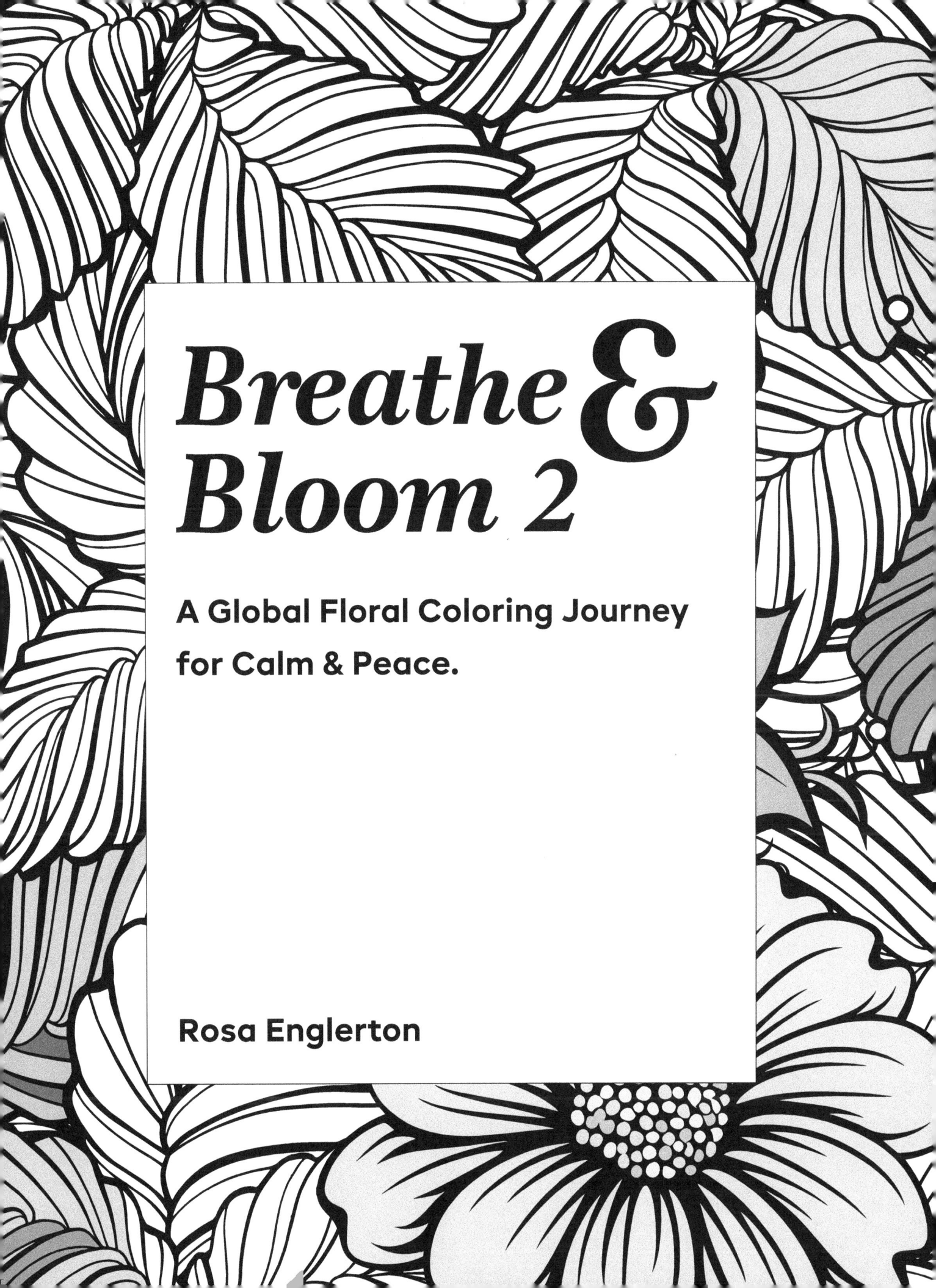

Breathe & Bloom 2

A Global Floral Coloring Journey for Calm & Peace.

Rosa Englerton

How to Use this Book

Hi and thank you for joining us in this journey of peace and relaxation.

This coloring book combines natural imagery with breathing exercises that help you return to return to ease and relaxation.

Help yourself affirms the right to rest and reset. Shifts your focus from being fixed to feeling free and elevated. Support yourself with mental clarity during chaotic moments. Reaffirm your will with agency during stress. Take a safe internal refuge. Restore your inner strength and balance.

The book has ten sections followed by ten-large size paintable flowers.

Start by reading the breathing exercise. Meditate on it for a few minutes, and start your breathing. Close your eyes. Look for the light of the Creator. Relax and put yourself in His hands.

Now you are ready to take your favourite coloring pencils, crayons, or markers, and let yourself flow into the flower and the colors. Be free. Imagine you are in the garden of Paradise. You are in control. The flower is your friend and is allowing you to give it the colors you want. Paint the background with patterns, or draw your own flowers.

When you are done painting, look at the flower, and do the breathing exercise again. If you have time, take a walk in the park. Look at the greenery, look at the flowers, see the colors in the world that surround you.

Breathe.

Everything is ok.
You are stronger now.

God Bless you!

Scent Imagination

Look at the flower on the opposite page.
- Close your eyes
- Imagine the scent of this flower
- Imagine its color

Cloud Thoughts

Sit quietly and imagine your thoughts as clouds drifting across the sky. Watch them come and go without clinging or pushing them away. Hang one of your worries to a cloud and blow them away.

Affirmation **Quote** *Calm is not a destination. It's a breath I return to.*

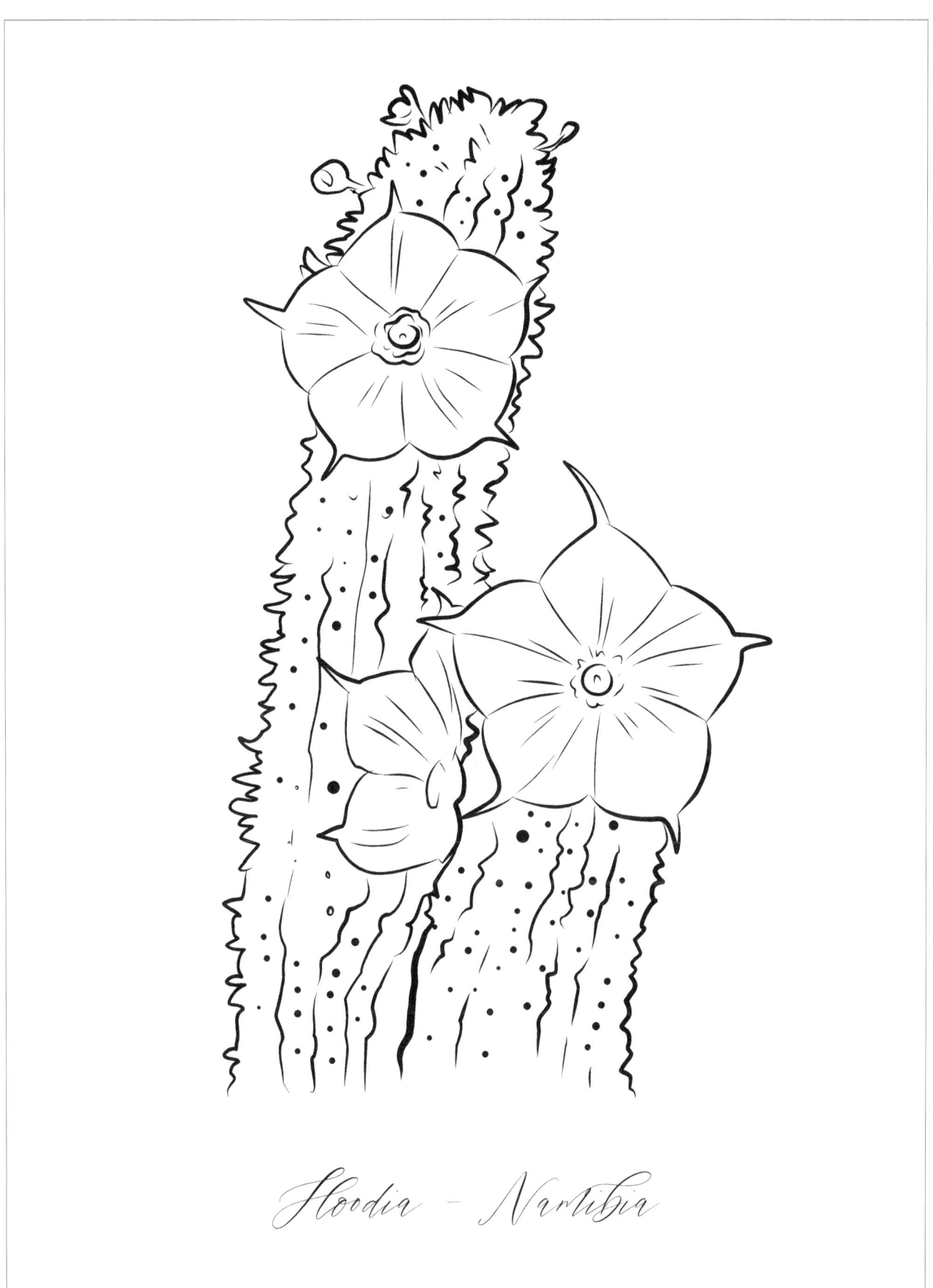

Hoodia - Namibia

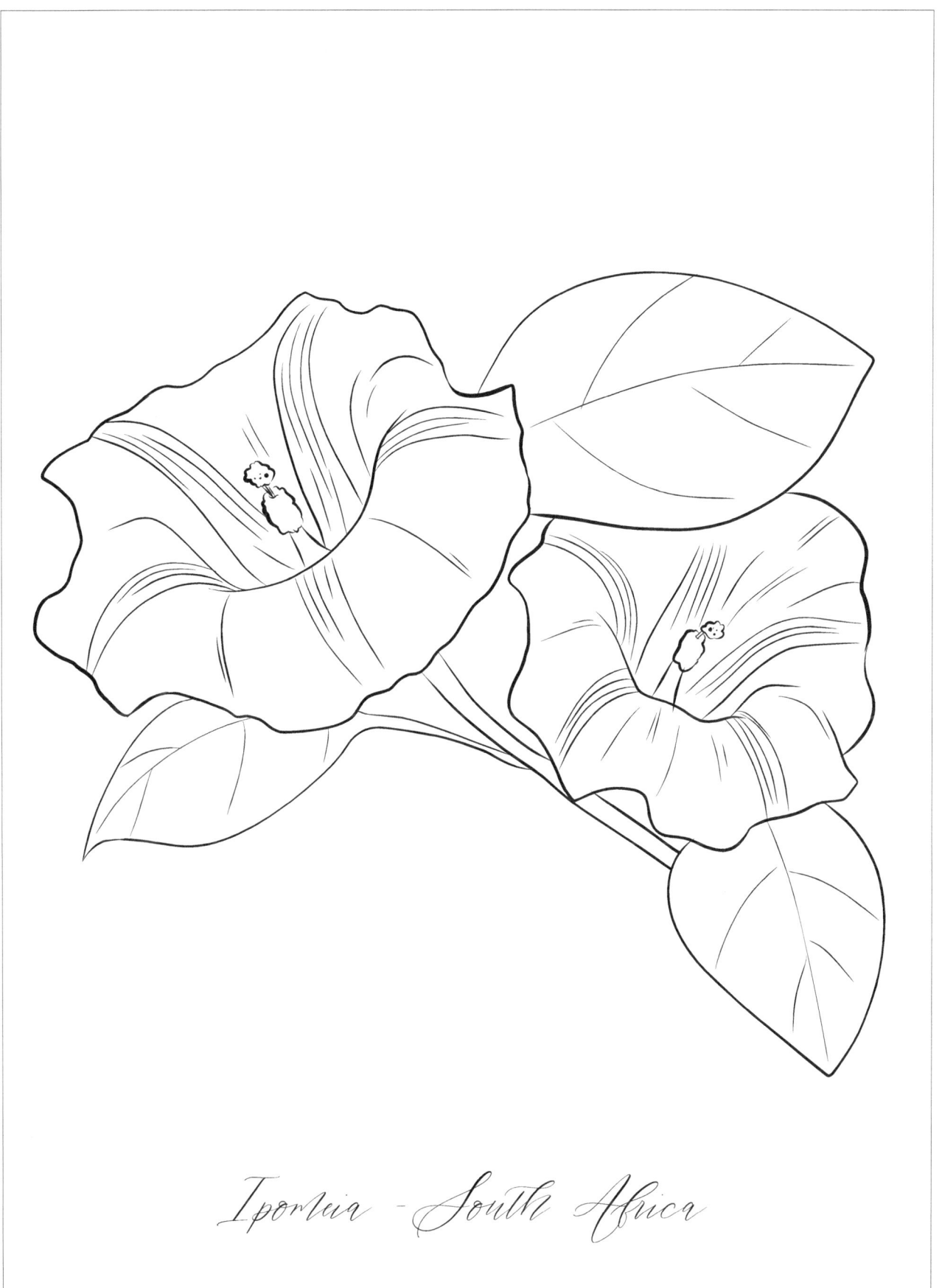

Ipomeia - South Africa

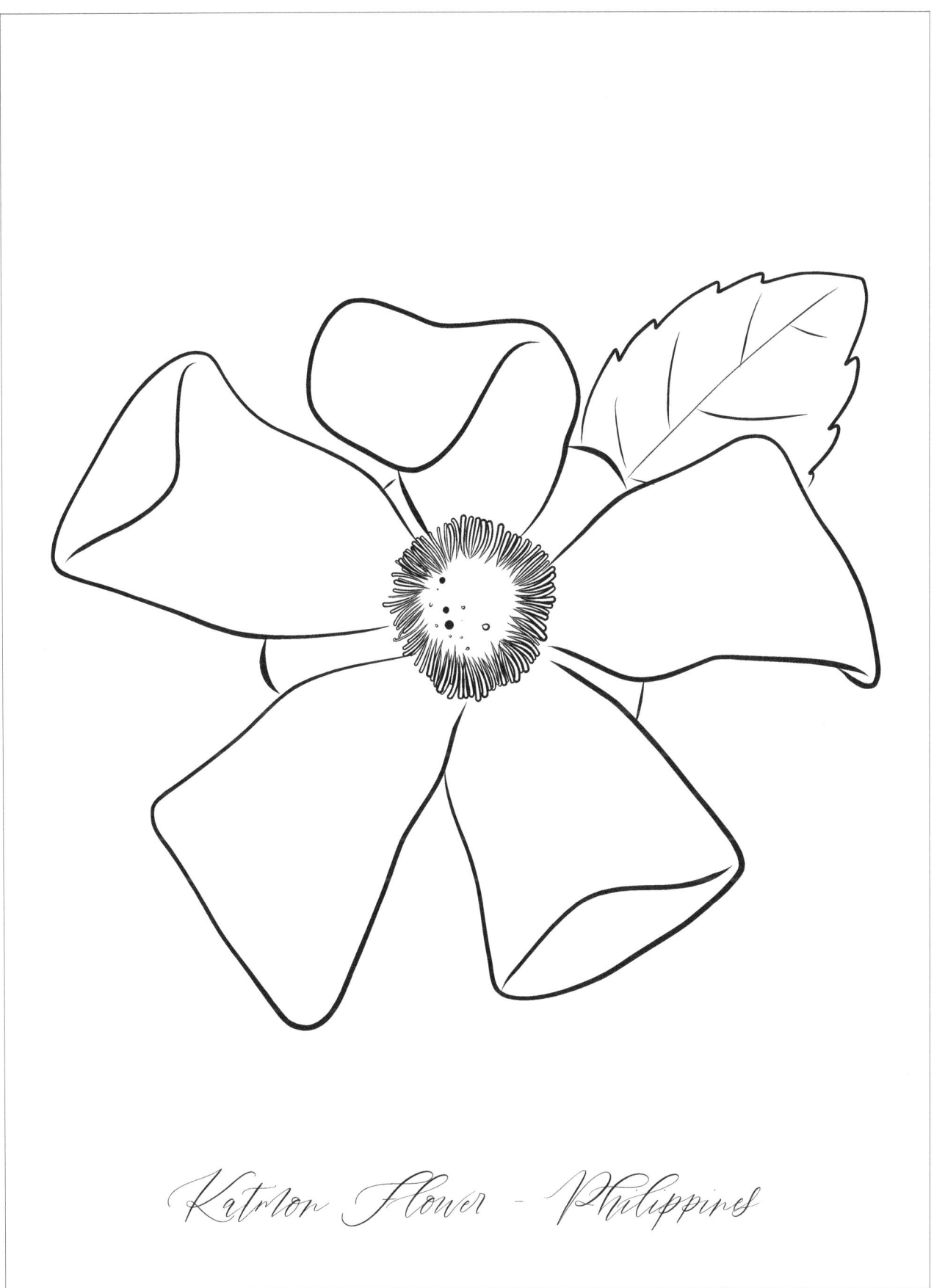

Katmon Flower - Philippines

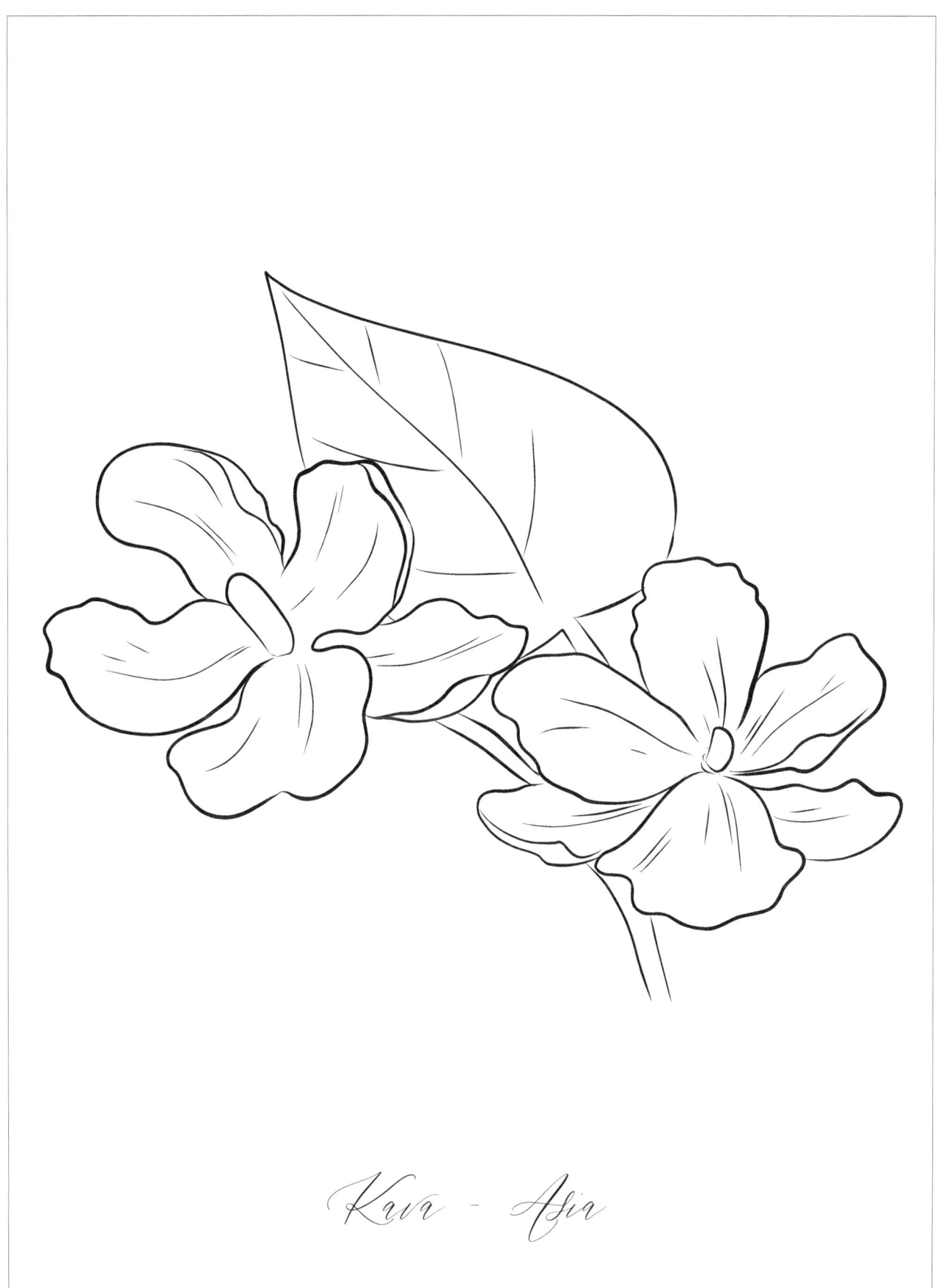

Kava - Asia

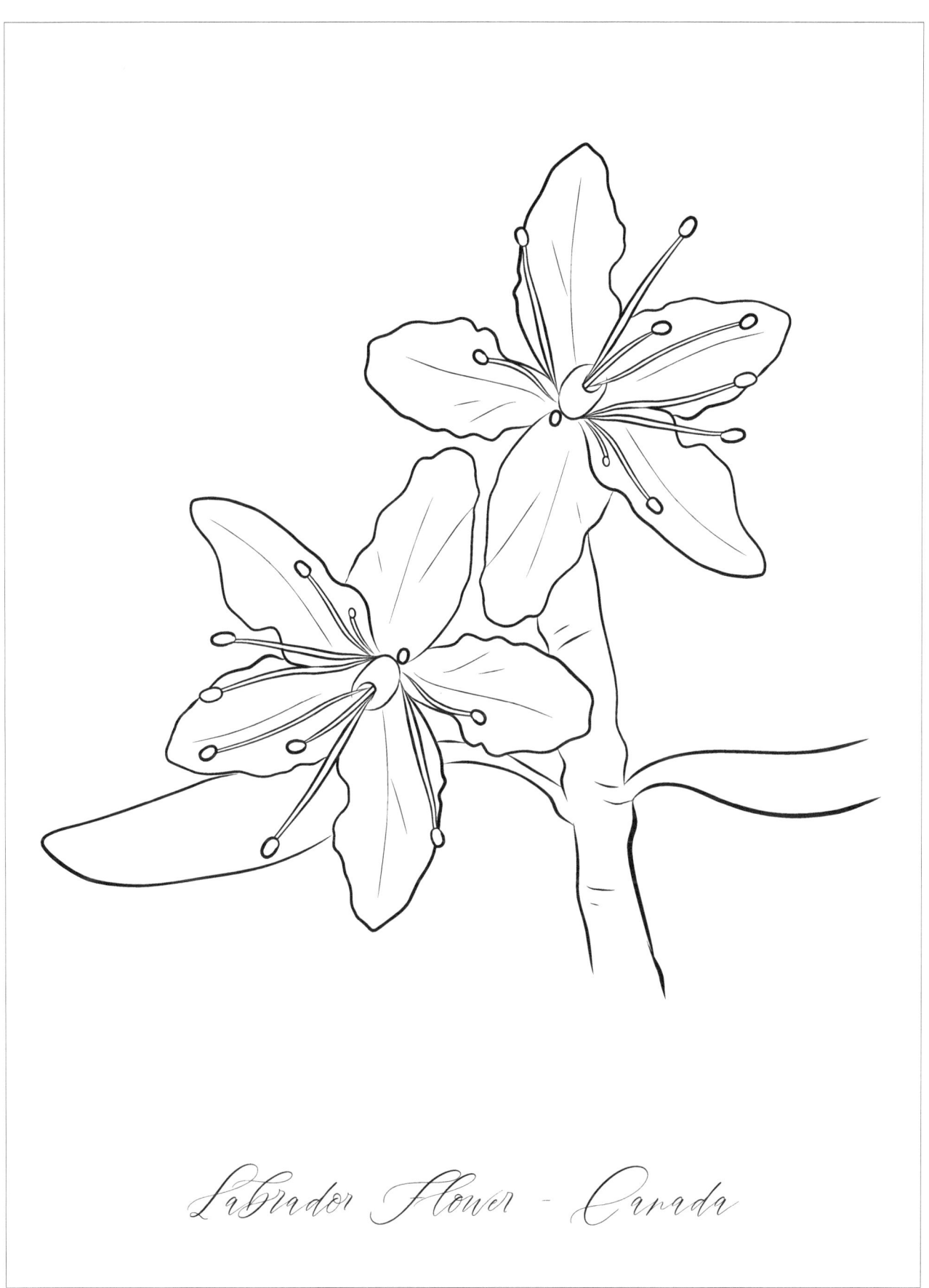

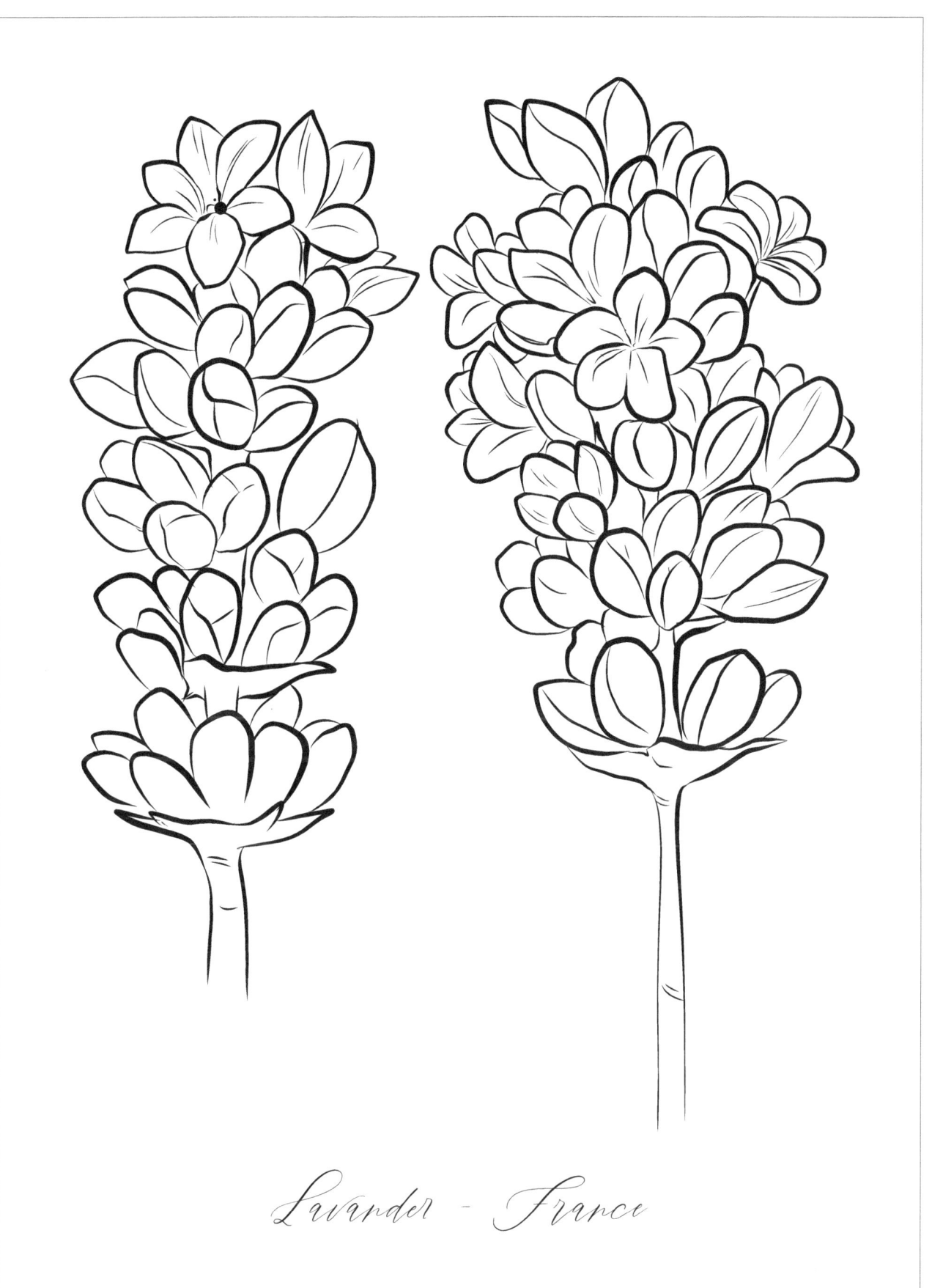

Lavander - France

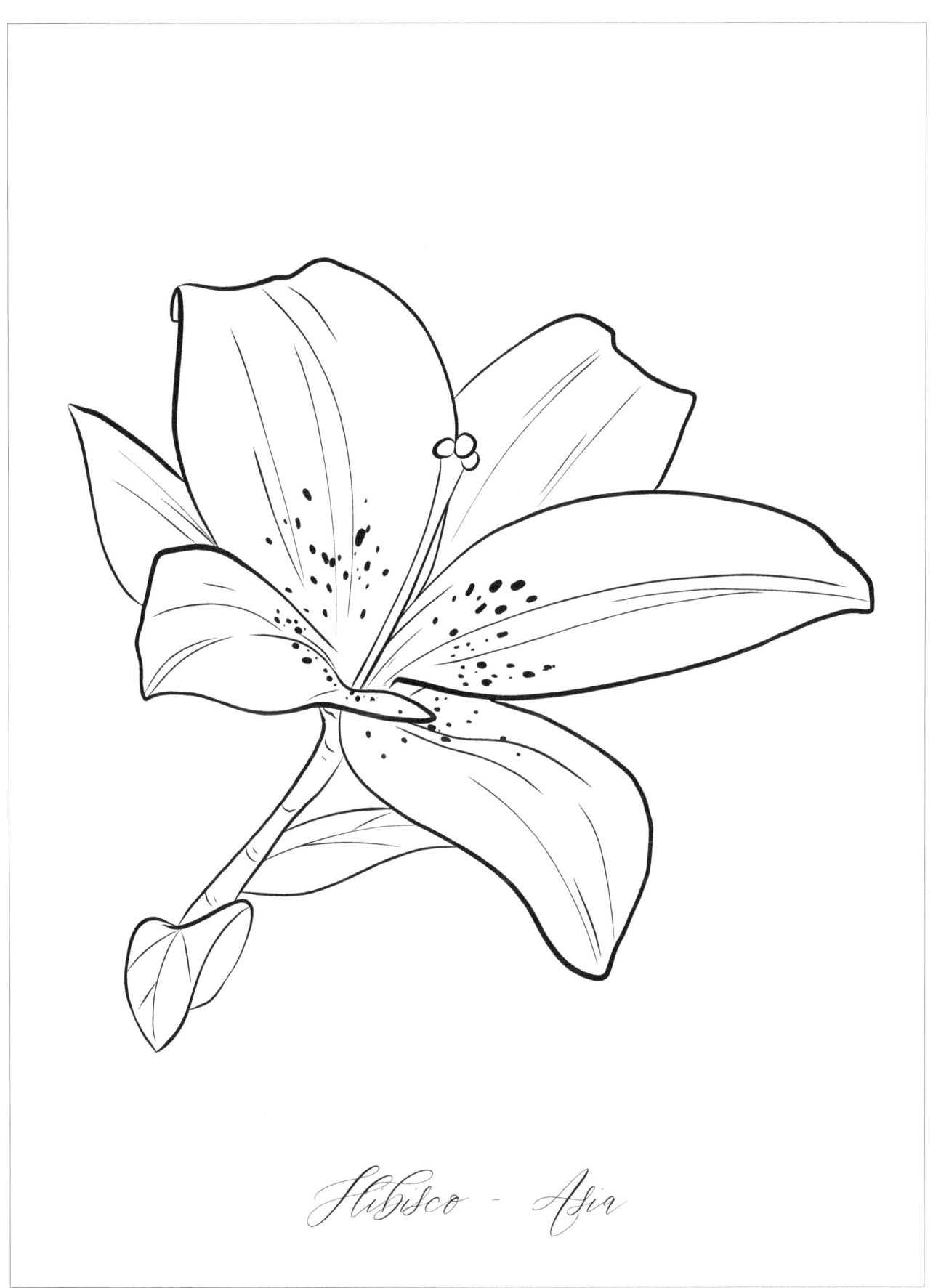

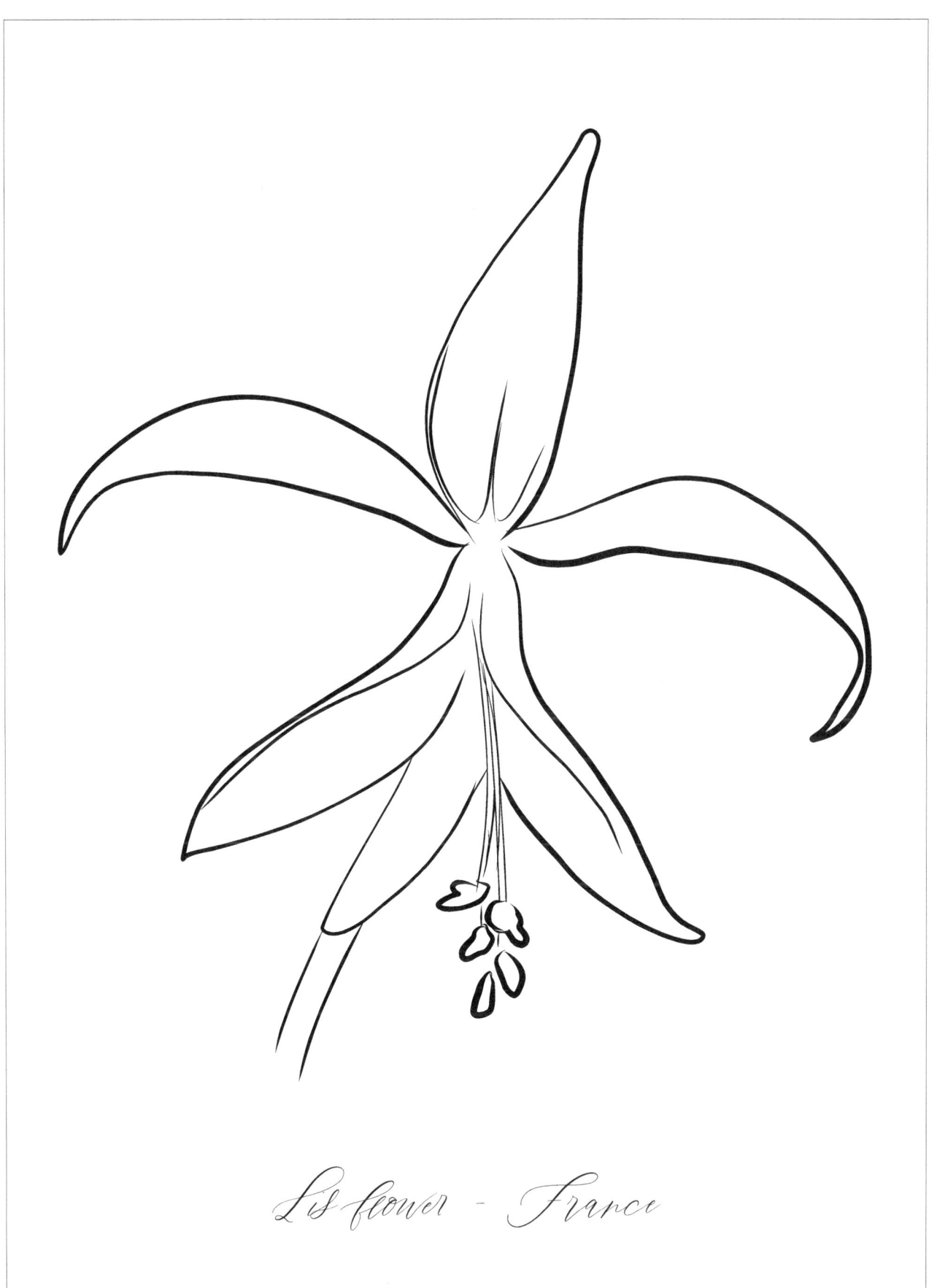

Lis flower - France

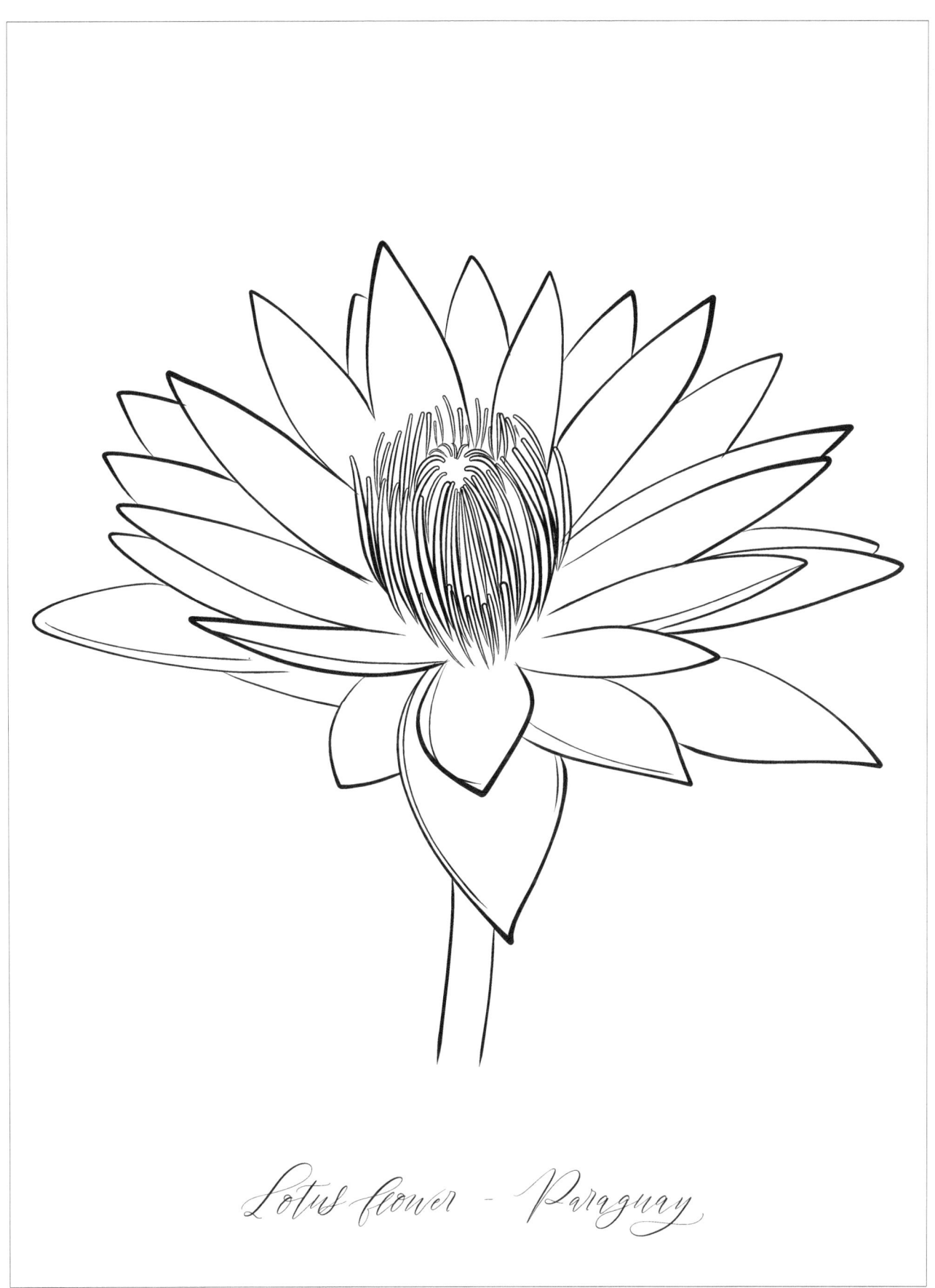

Lotus flower - Paraguay

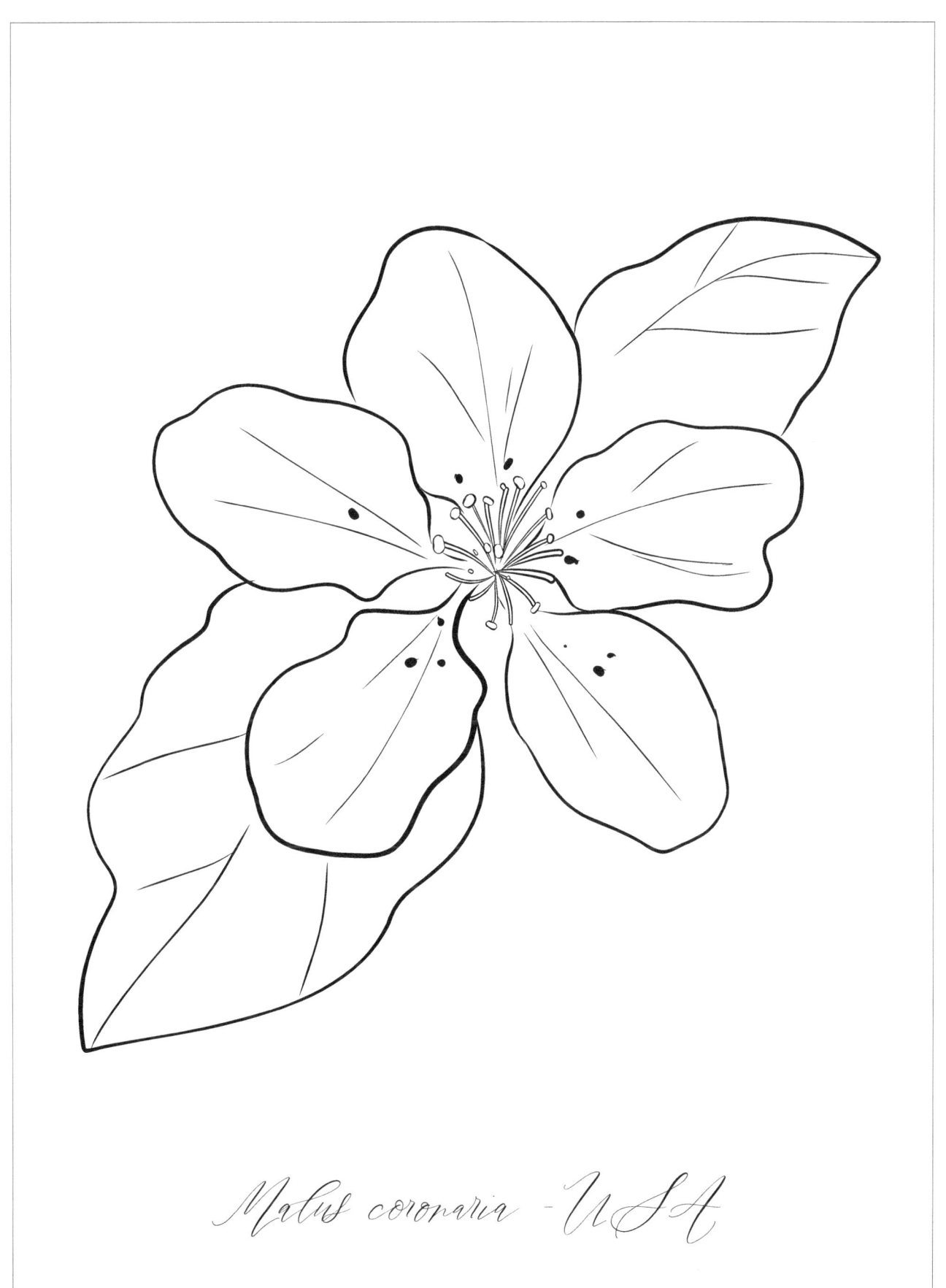

Malus coronaria - USA

Scent Imagination

Look at the flower on the opposite page.
- Close your eyes
- Imagine the scent of this flower
- Imagine its color

Flower in Your Palm

Imagine holding a flower in your palm. Feel its weight, texture, and softness. It silky like your skin. Inhale slowly. Smelling its scent, and exhale gently.

Affirmation **Quote**

I breathe in clarity.
I breathe out the noise.

I breath in freedom,
I breath out pain.

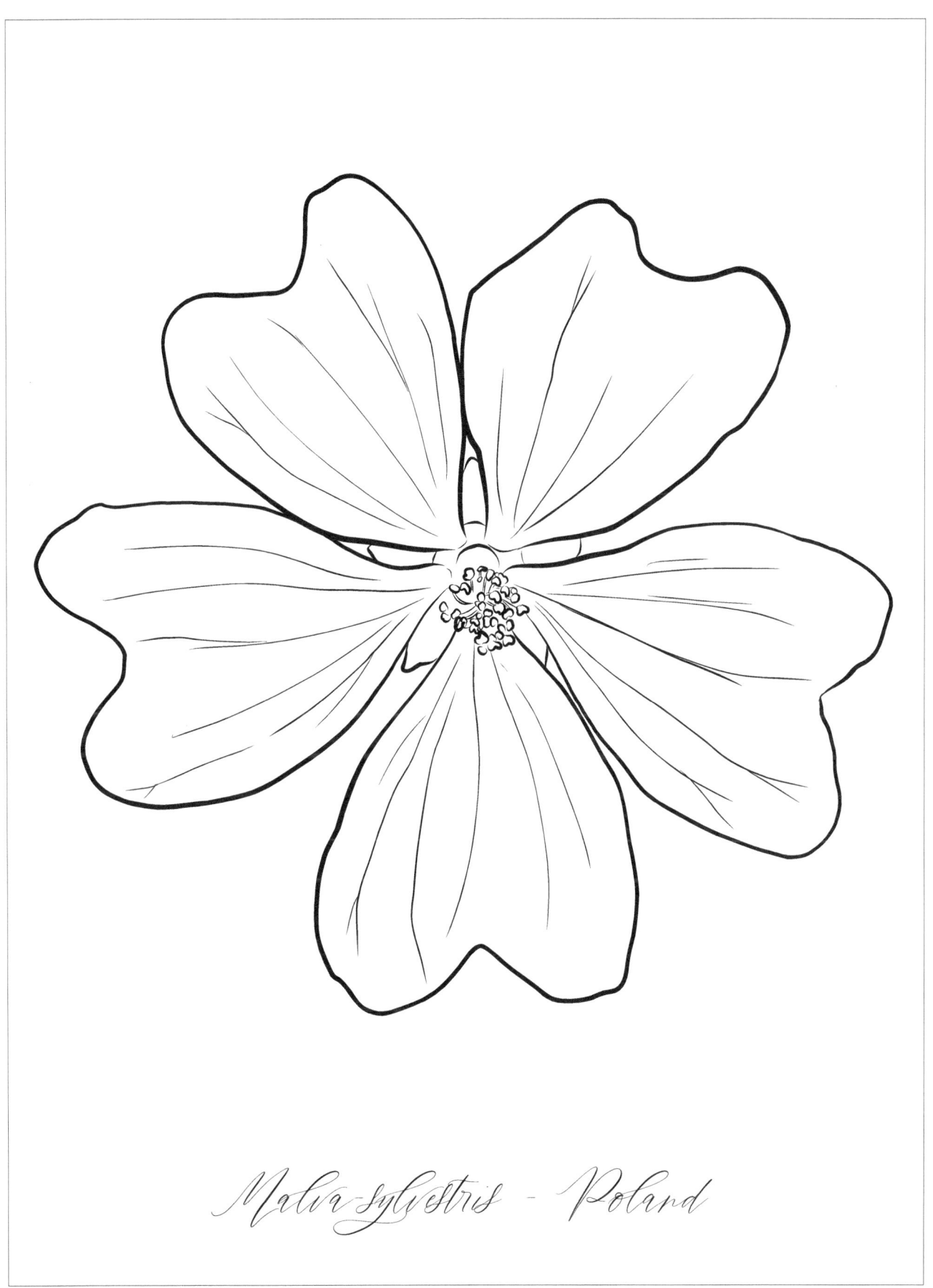

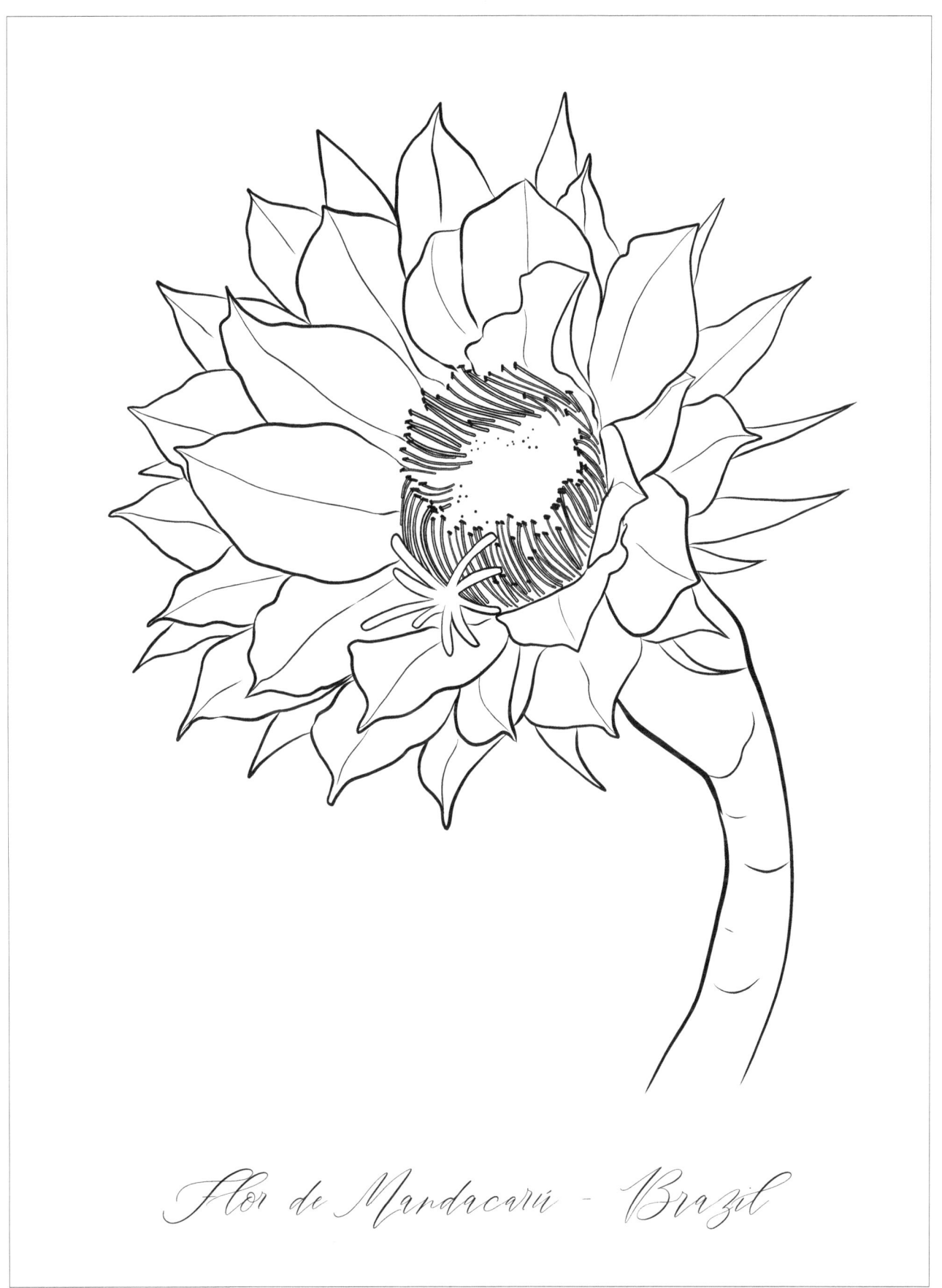

Flor de Mandacaru - Brazil

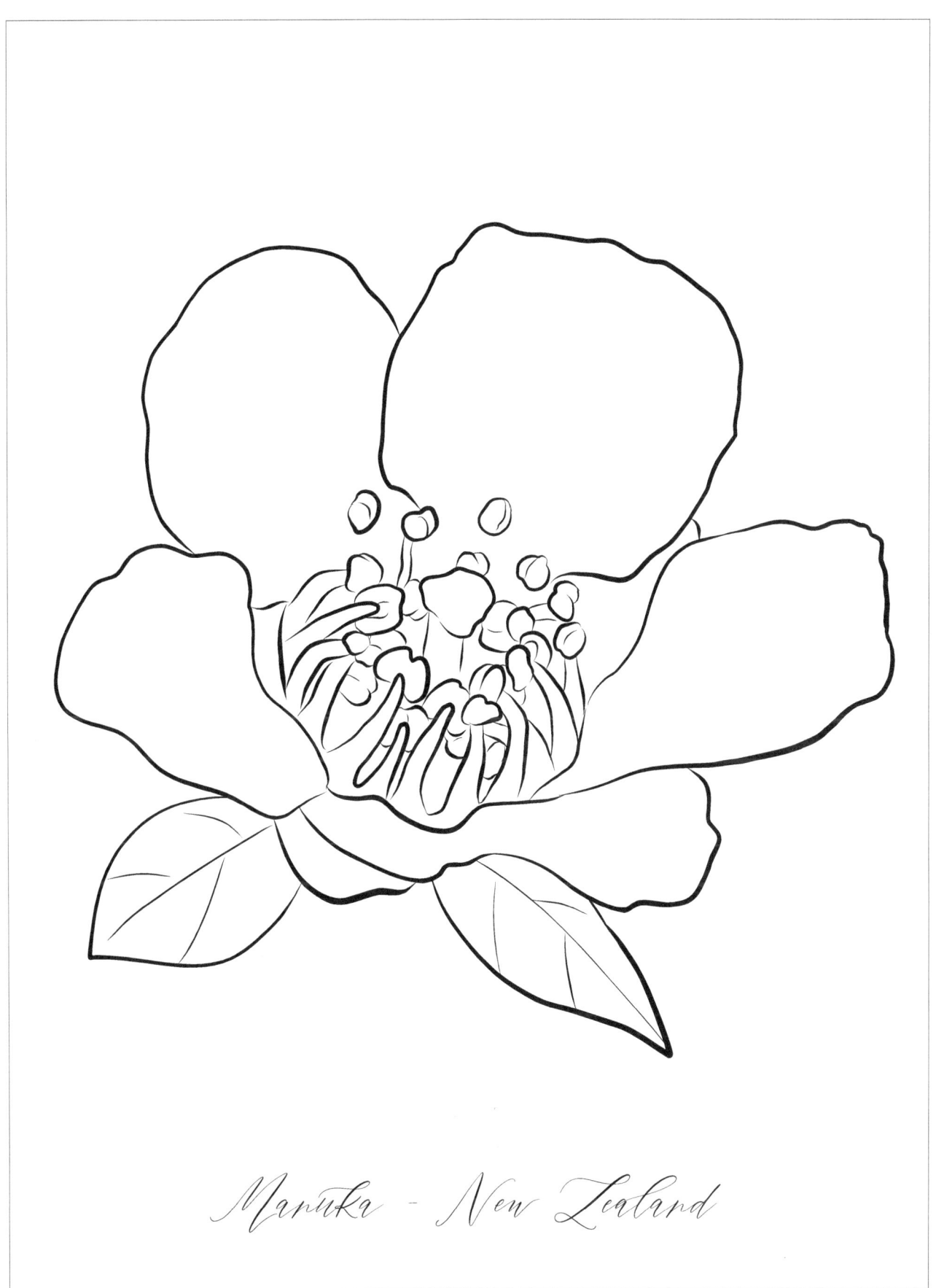

Manuka - New Zealand

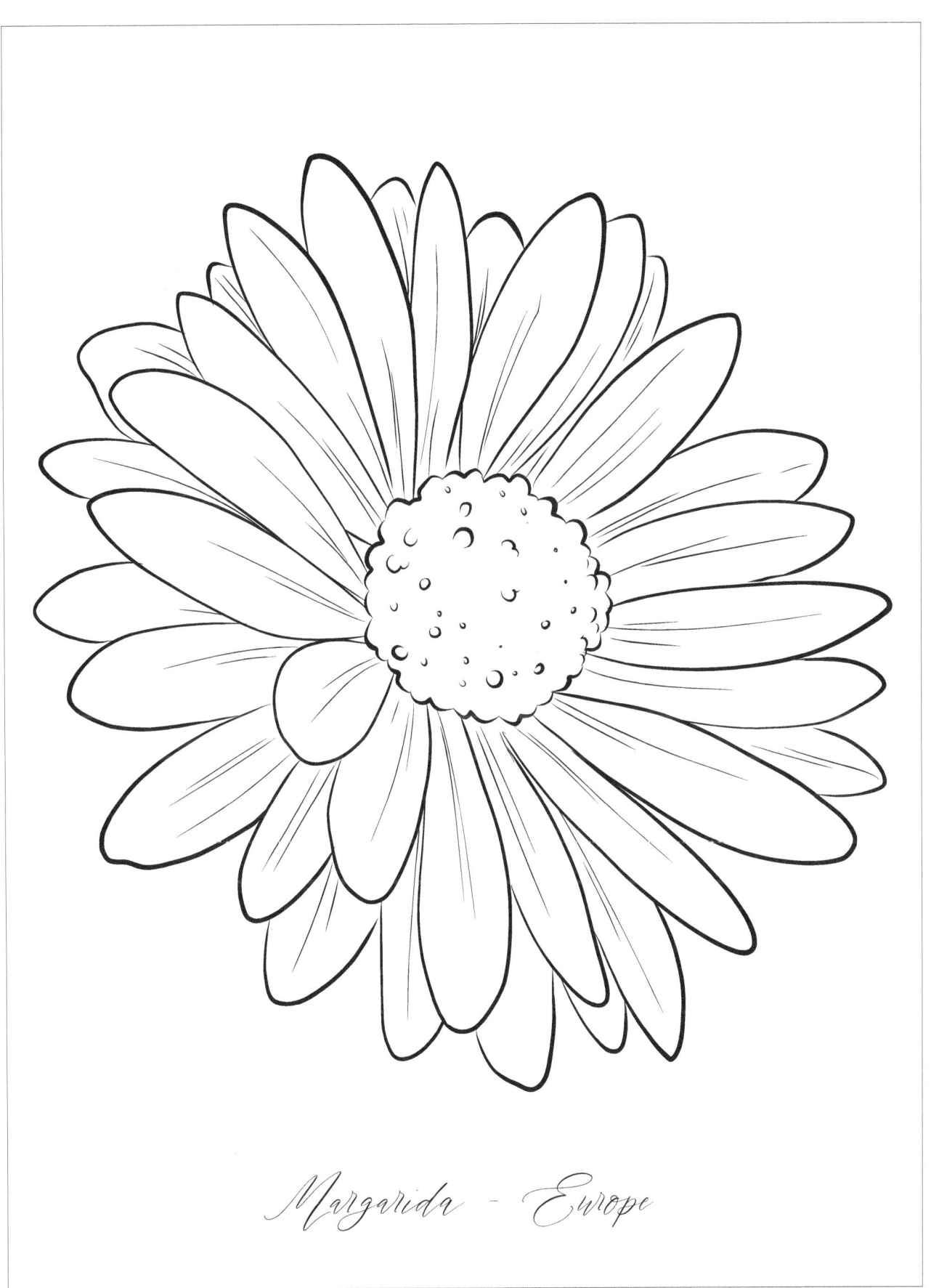

Margarida – Europe

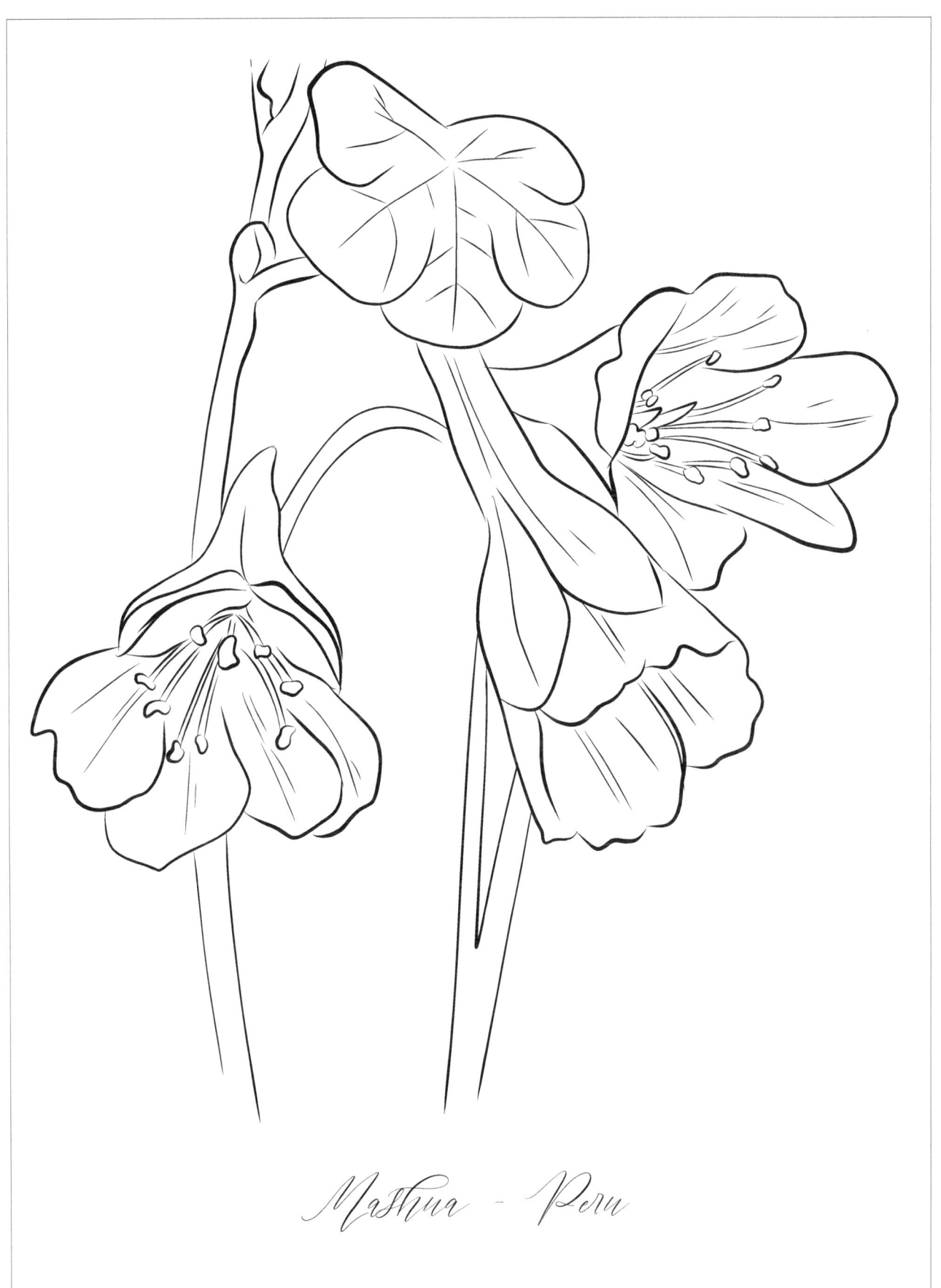

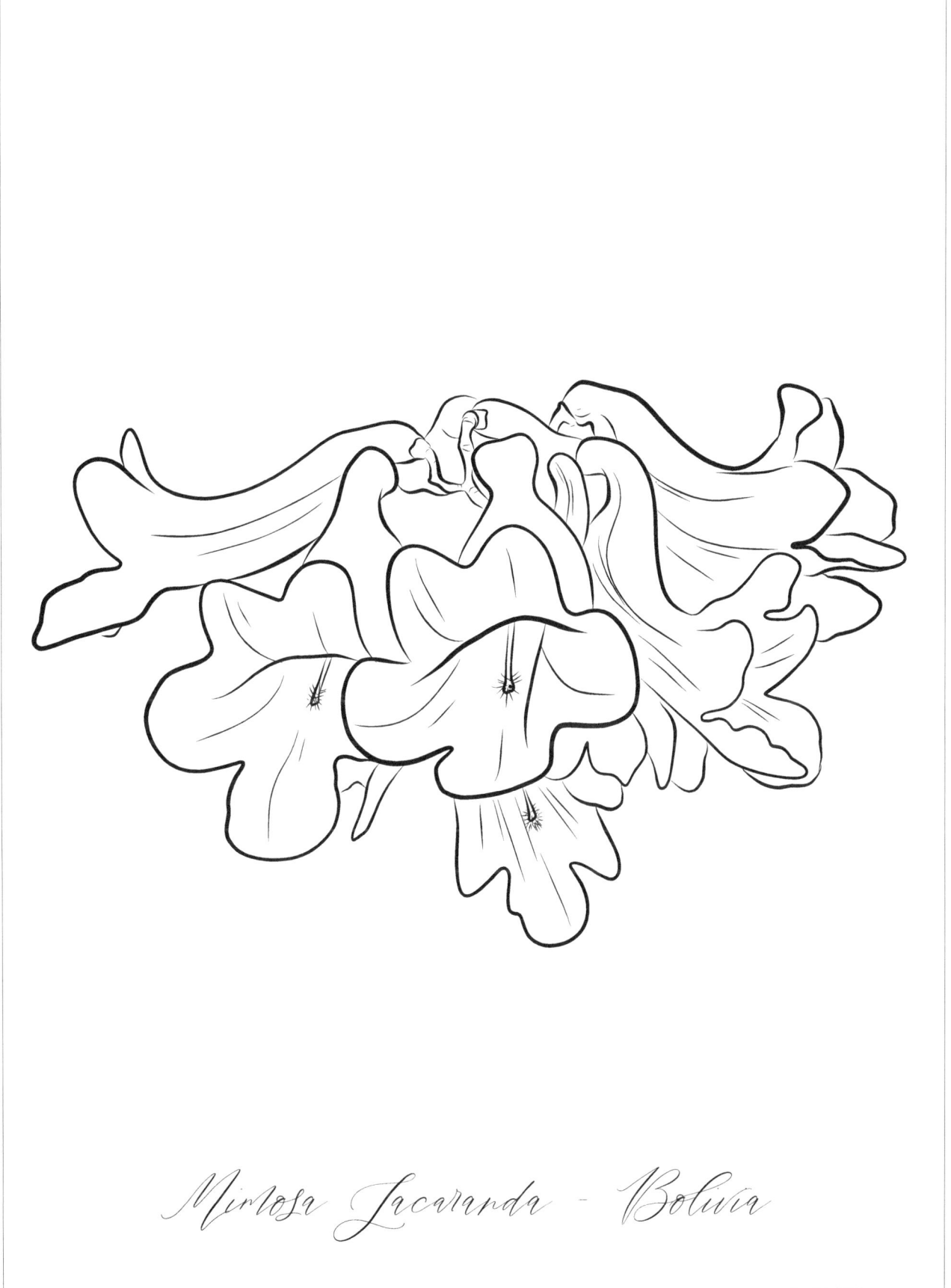

Mimosa Jacaranda - Bolivia

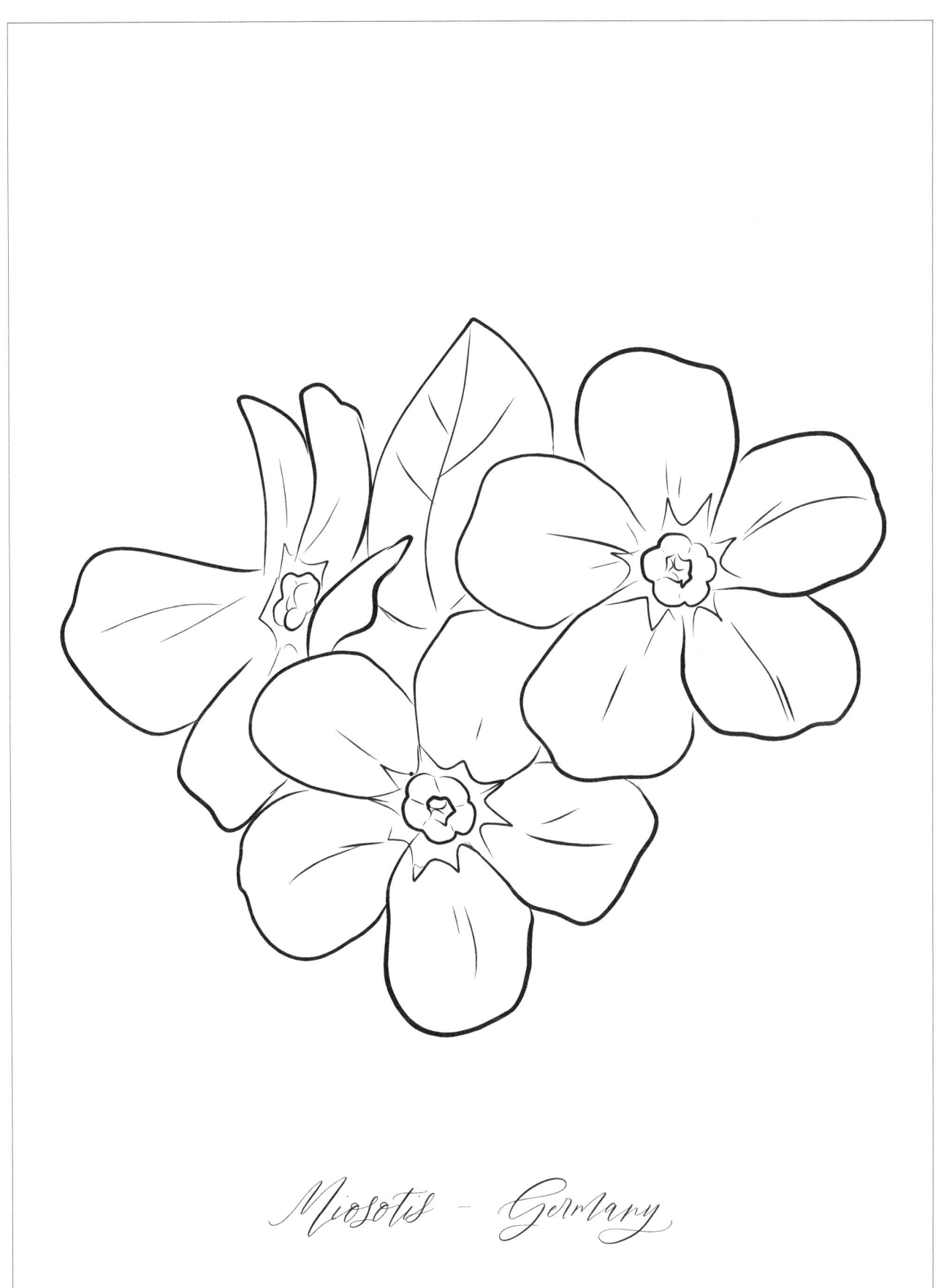

Miosotis – Germany

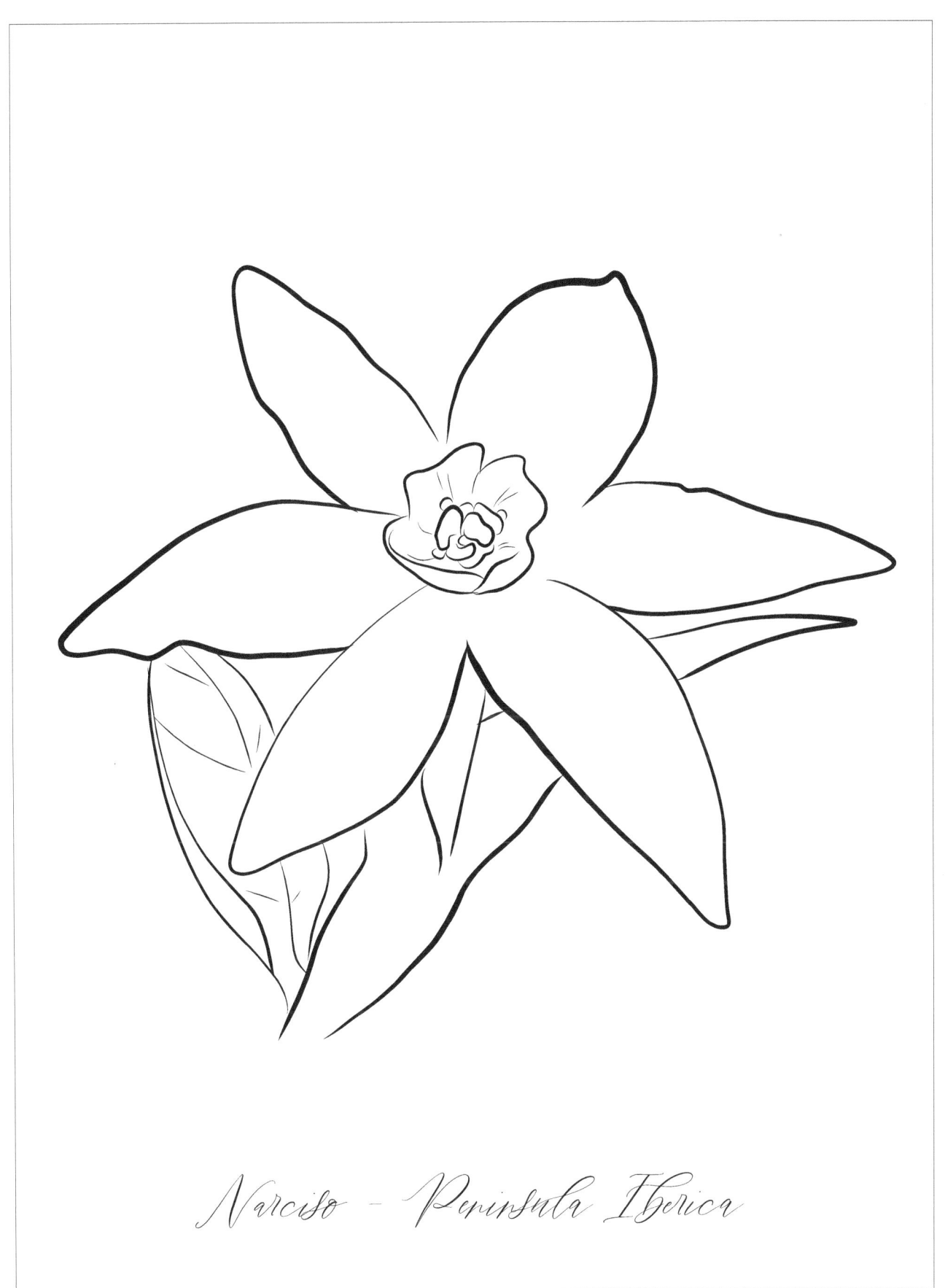

Narciso - Peninsula Iberica

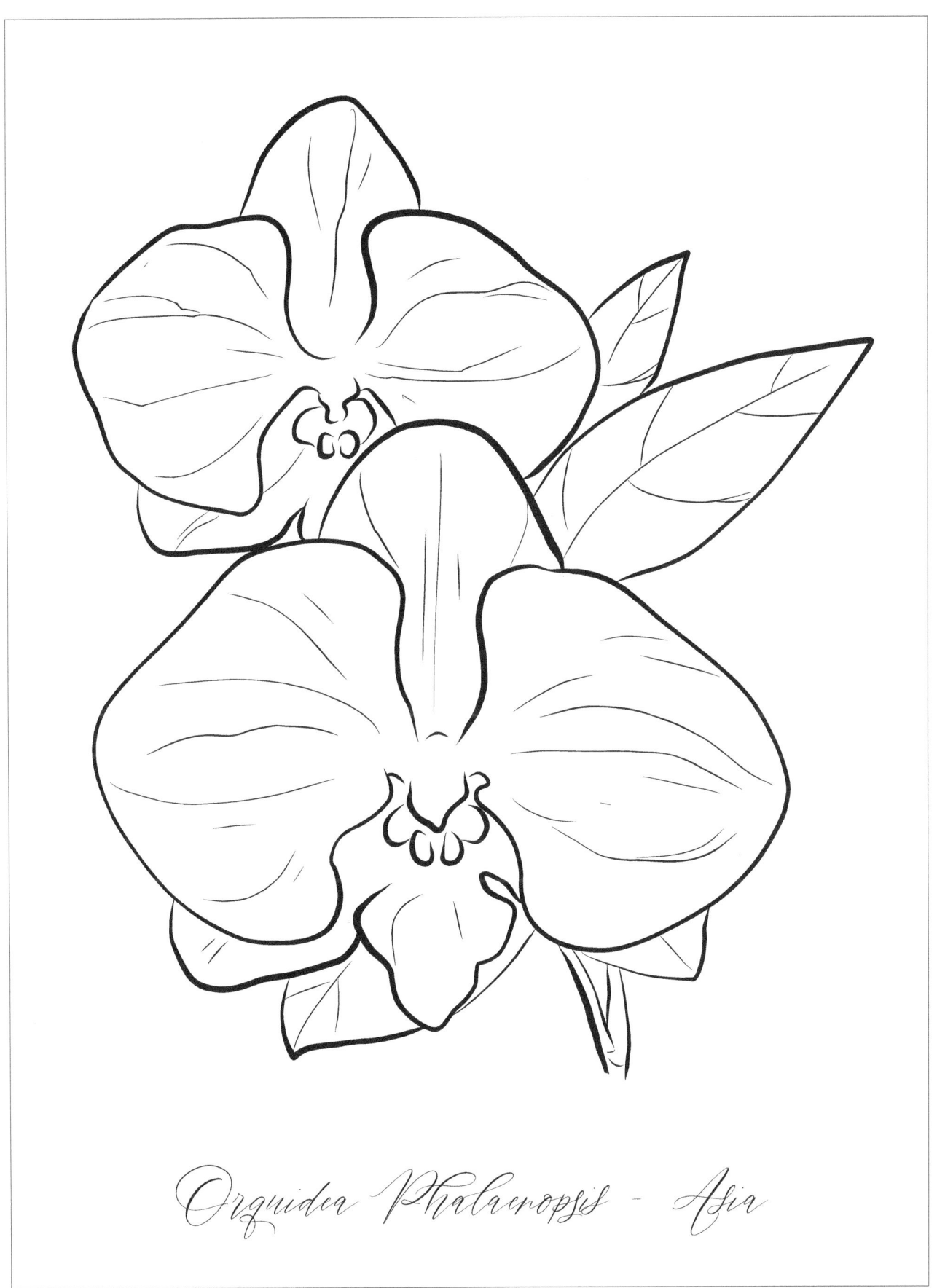

Orquidea Phalaenopsis - Asia

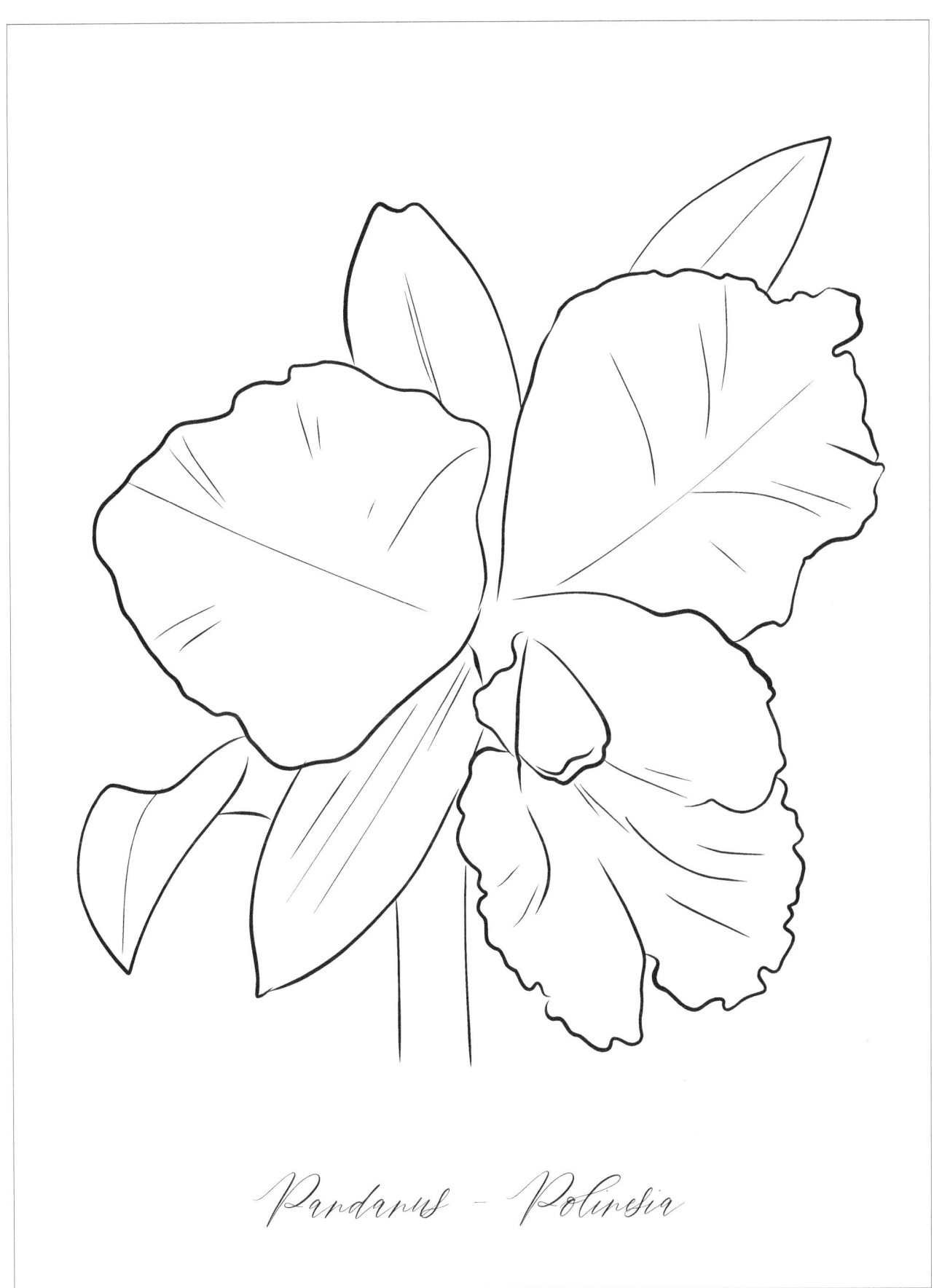

Pandanus - Polinesia

Scent Imagination

Look at the flower on the opposite page.

- Close your eyes
- Imagine the scent of this flower
- Imagine its color

The Reset Breath

Take one deep inhale (through the nose), hold for 2 seconds, and exhale with a long sigh. Do this just, intentionally. When you exhale, push out that worry. Push out that pain. Inhale the pure scent of Paradise.

Affirmation Quote

Even now, I can choose stillness.

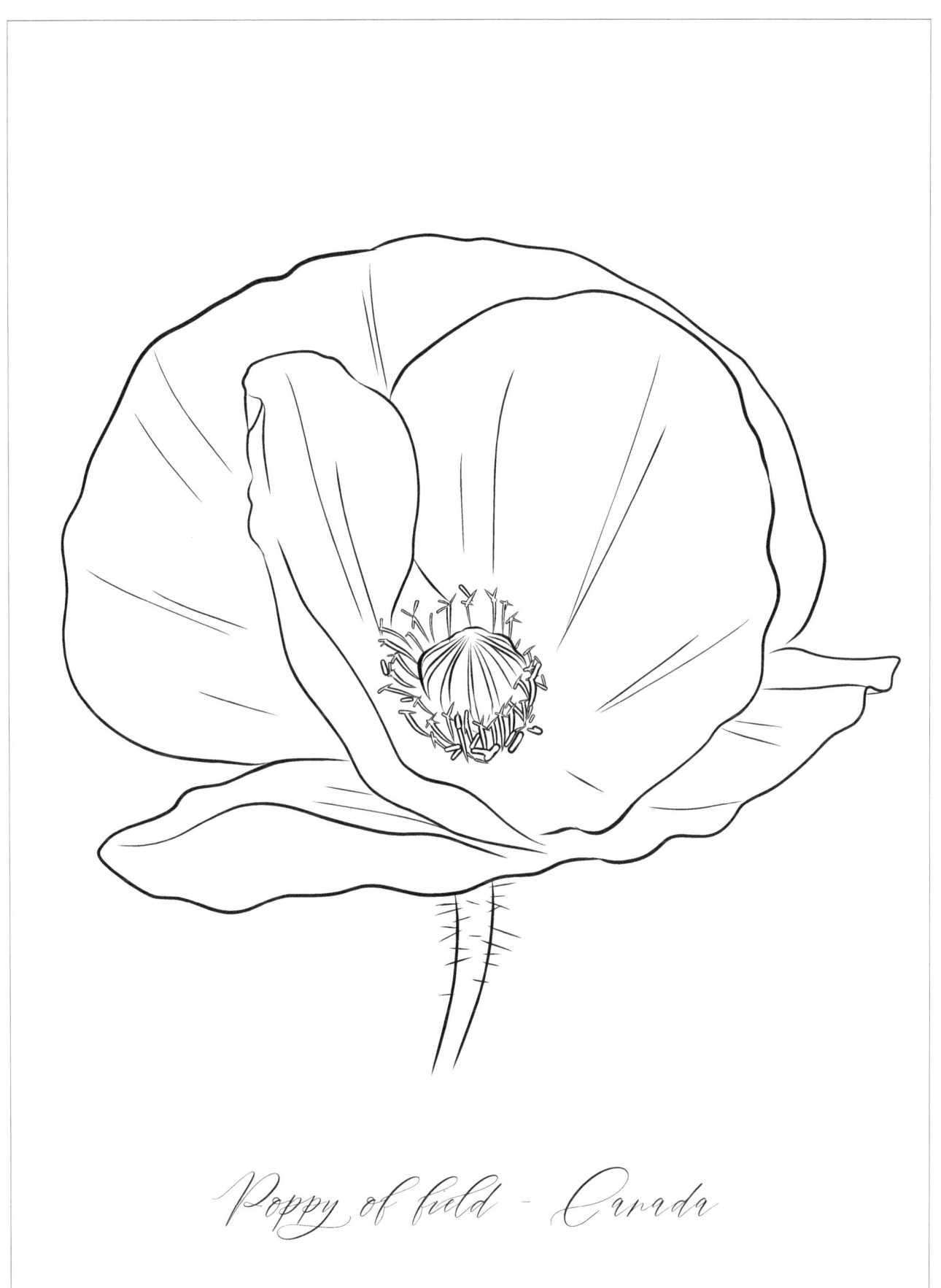

Poppy of field - Canada

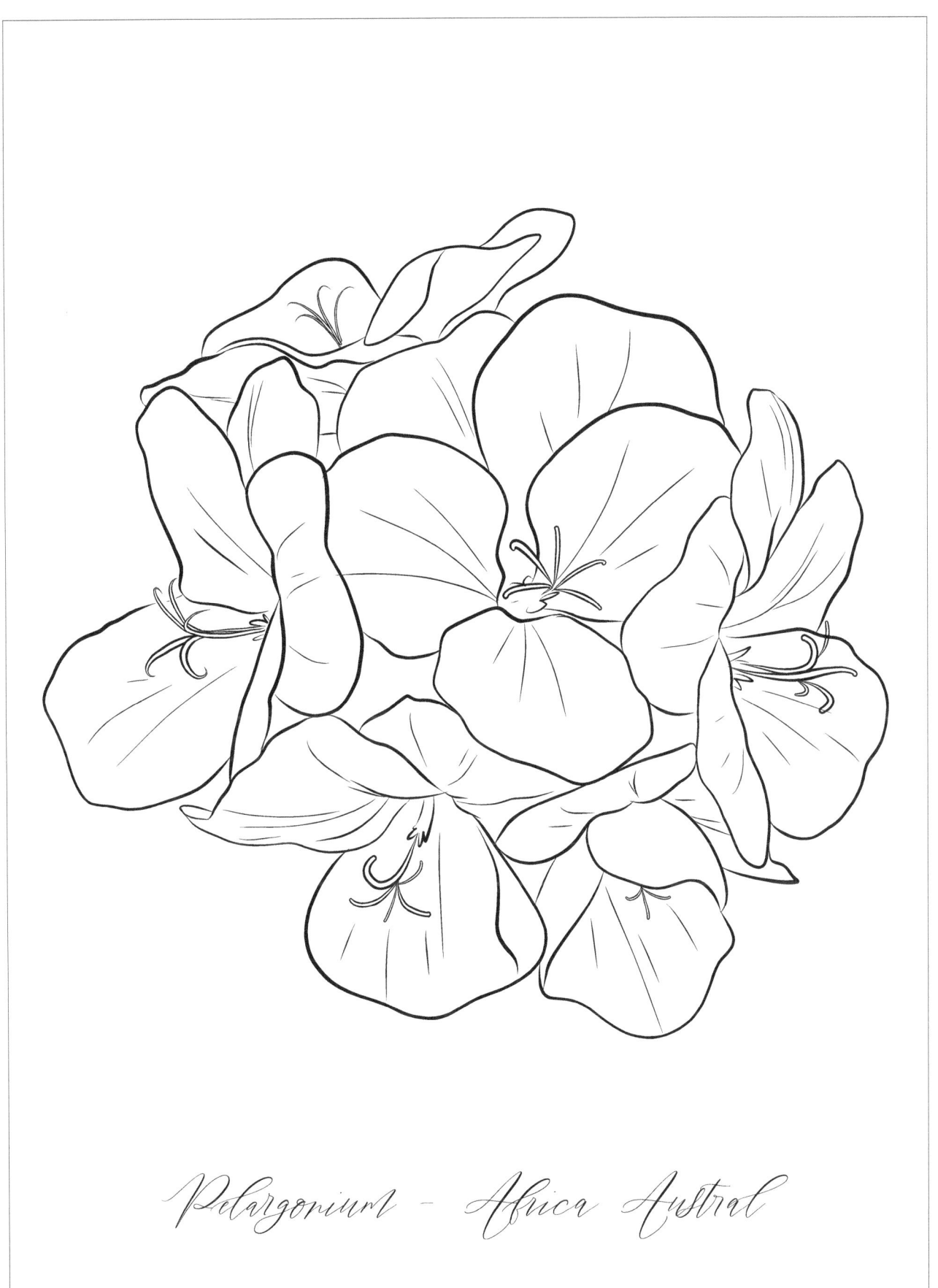

Pelargonium – Africa Austral

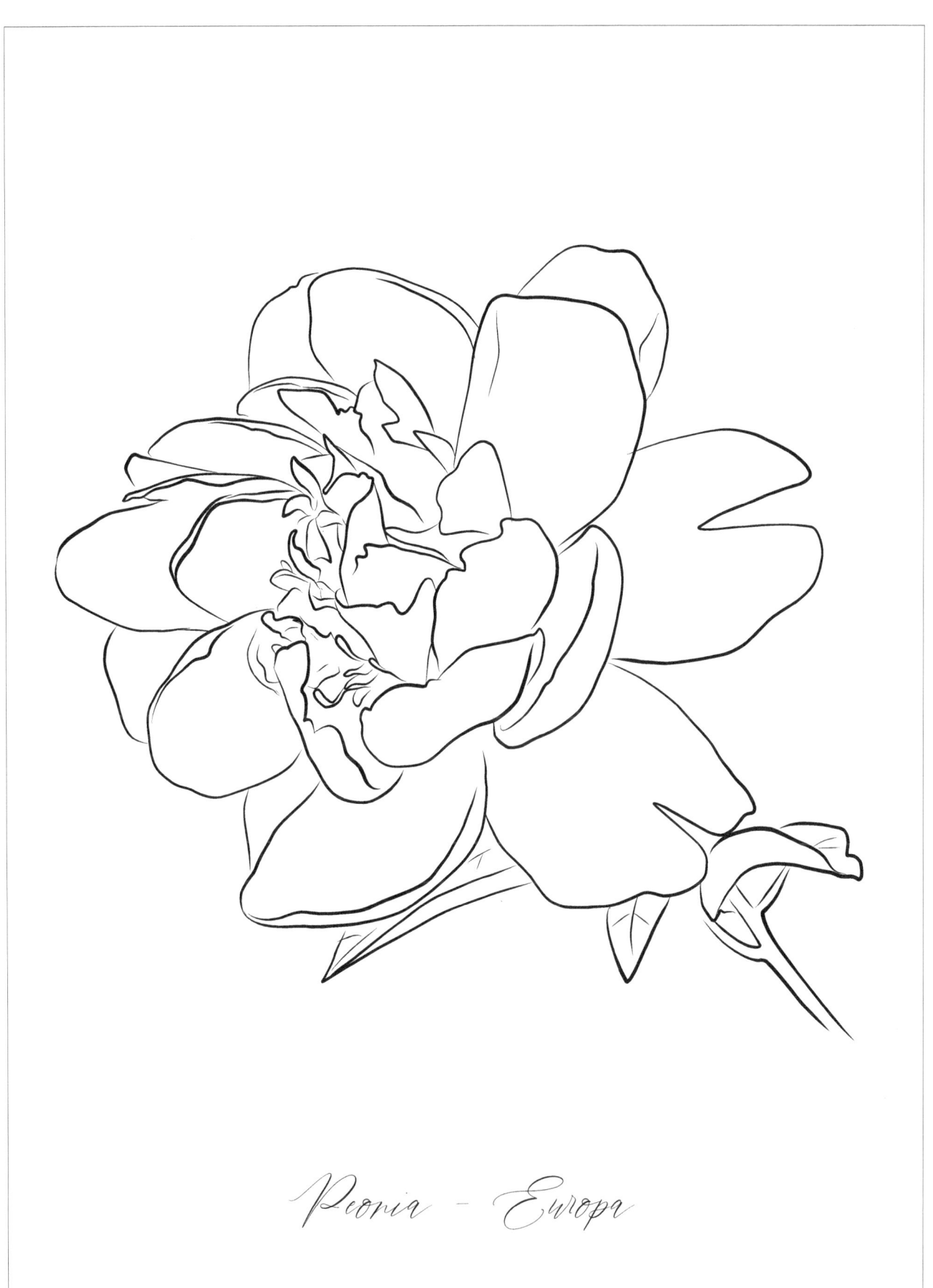

Peonia - Europa

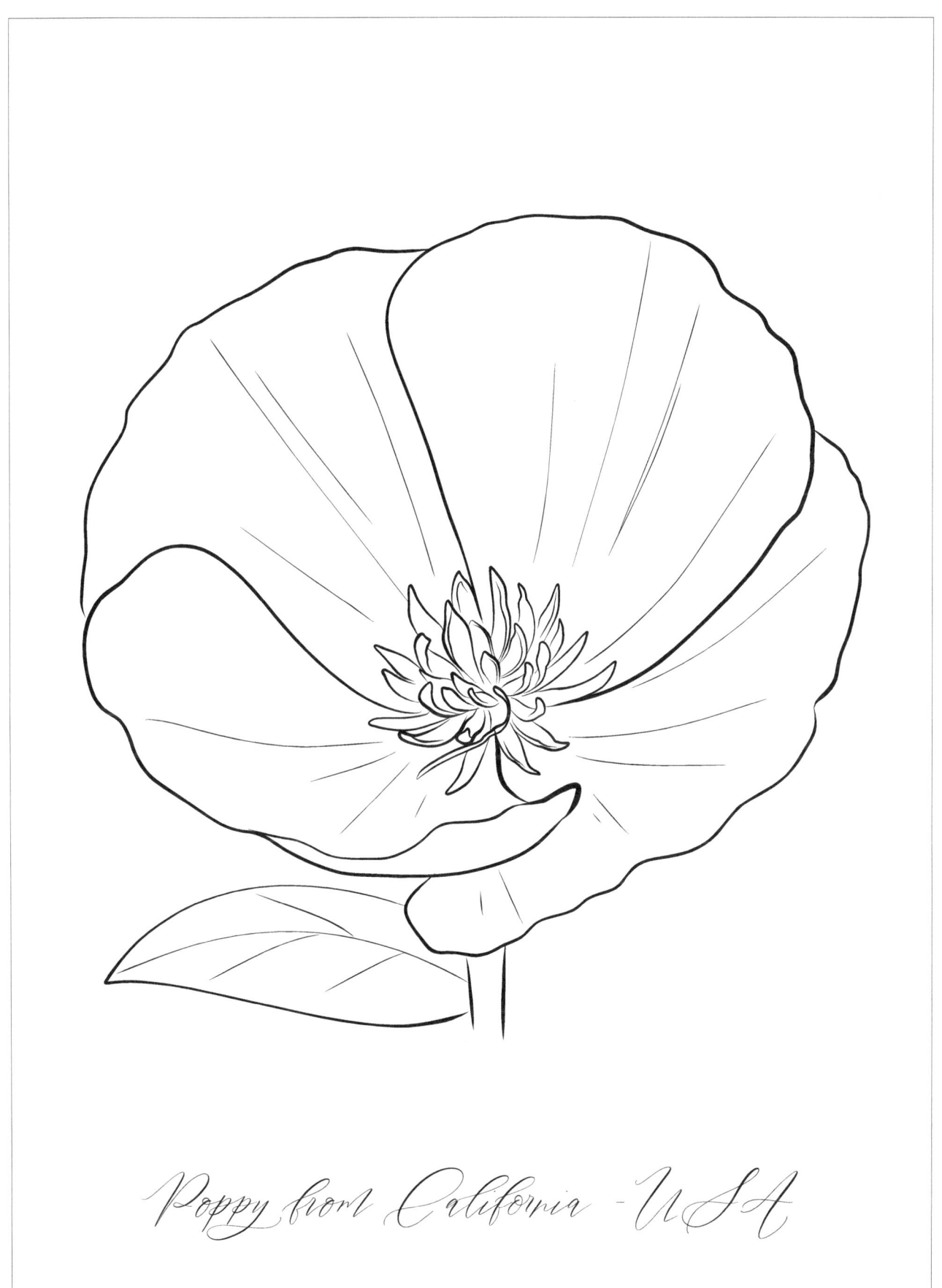

Poppy from California - USA

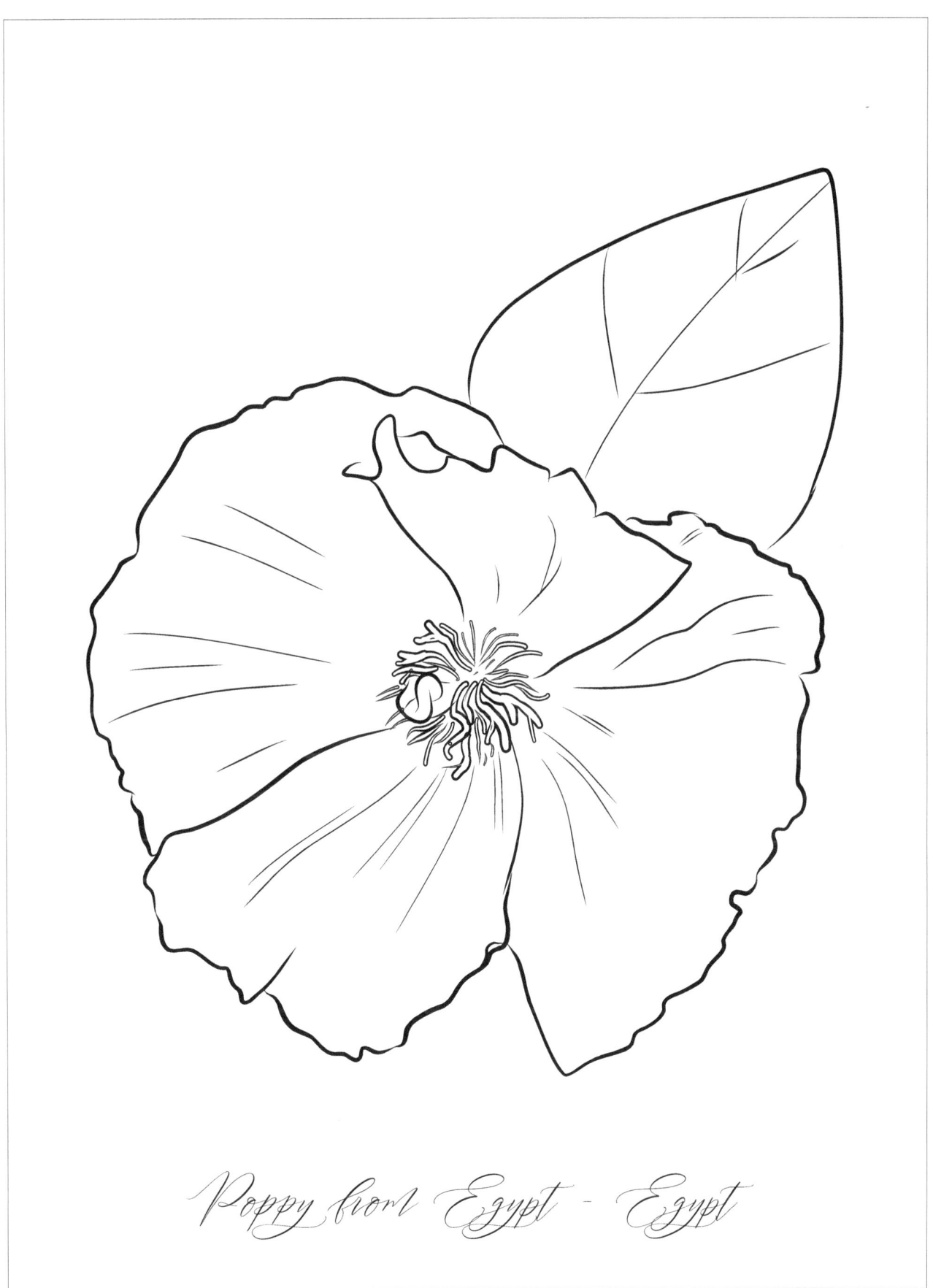

Poppy from Egypt - Egypt

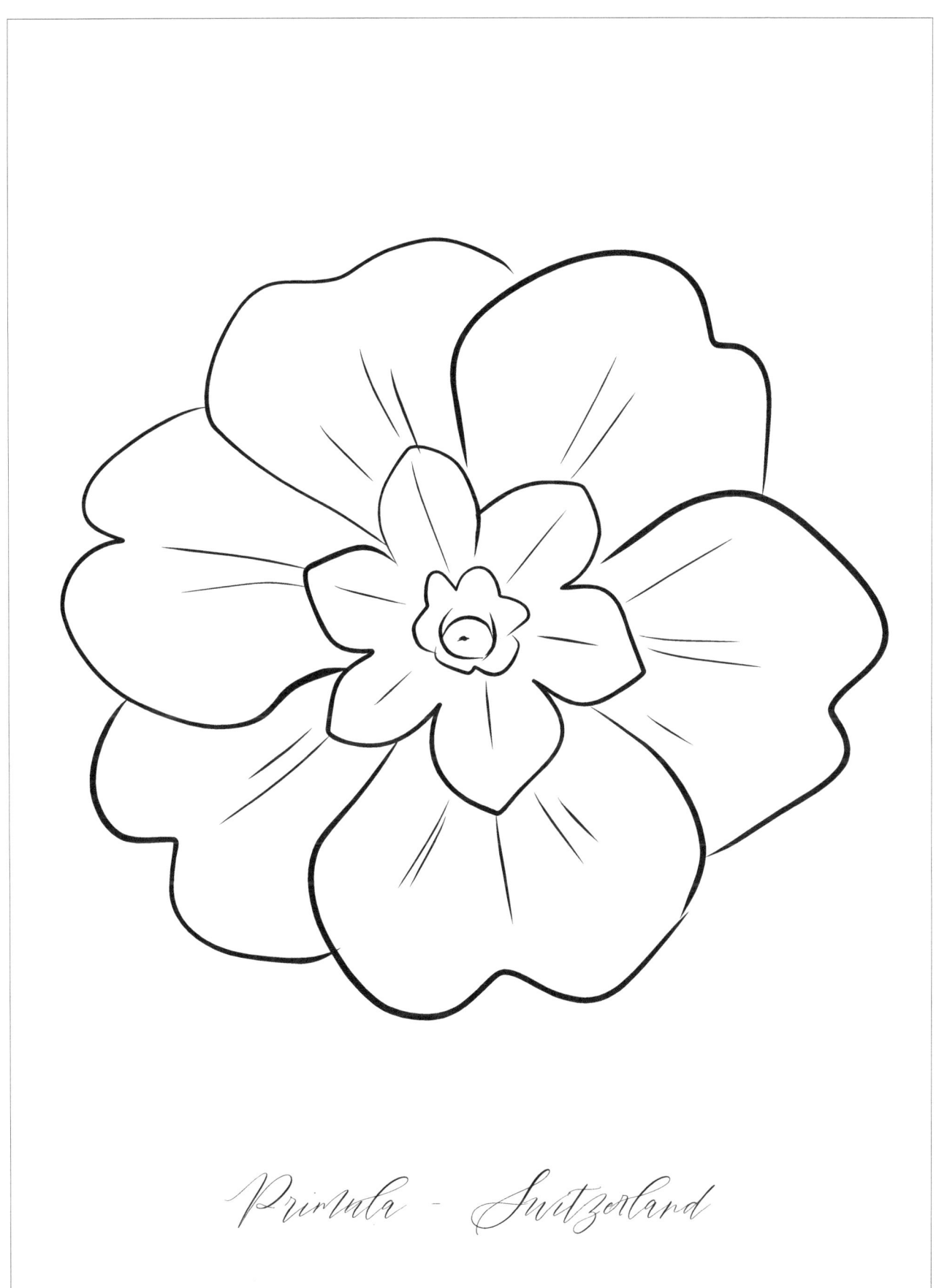

Primula – Switzerland

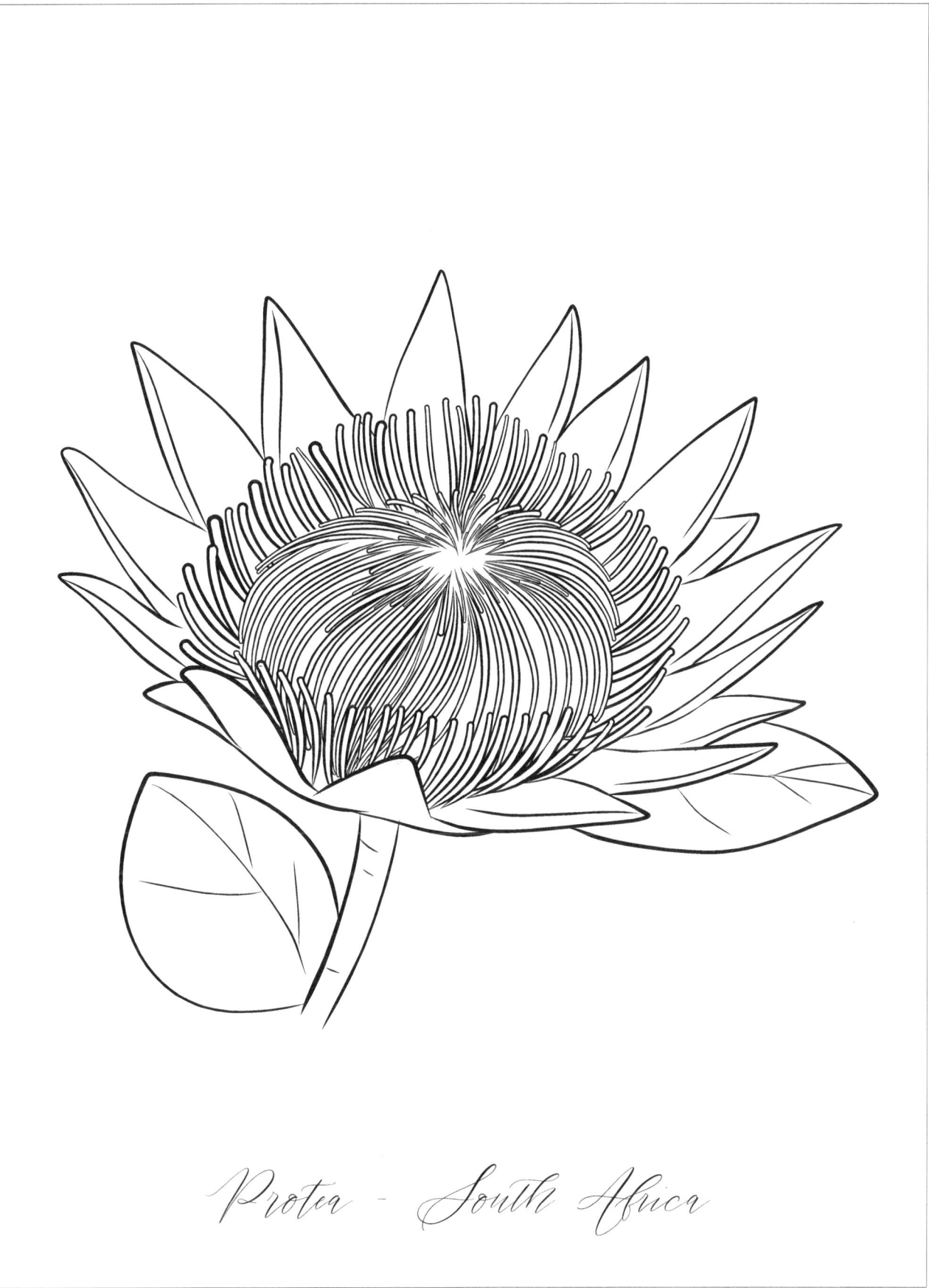

Protea - South Africa

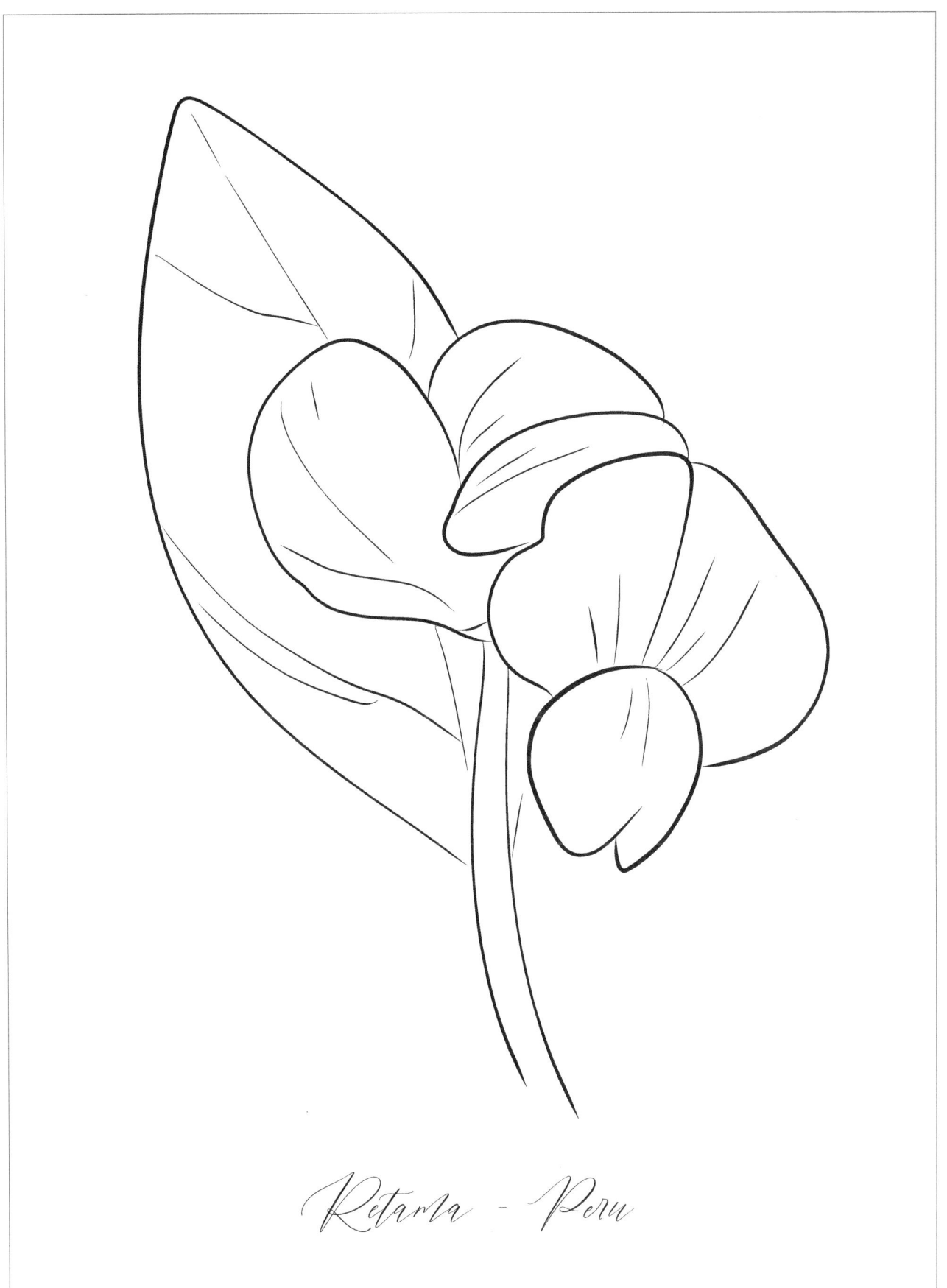

Retama - Peru

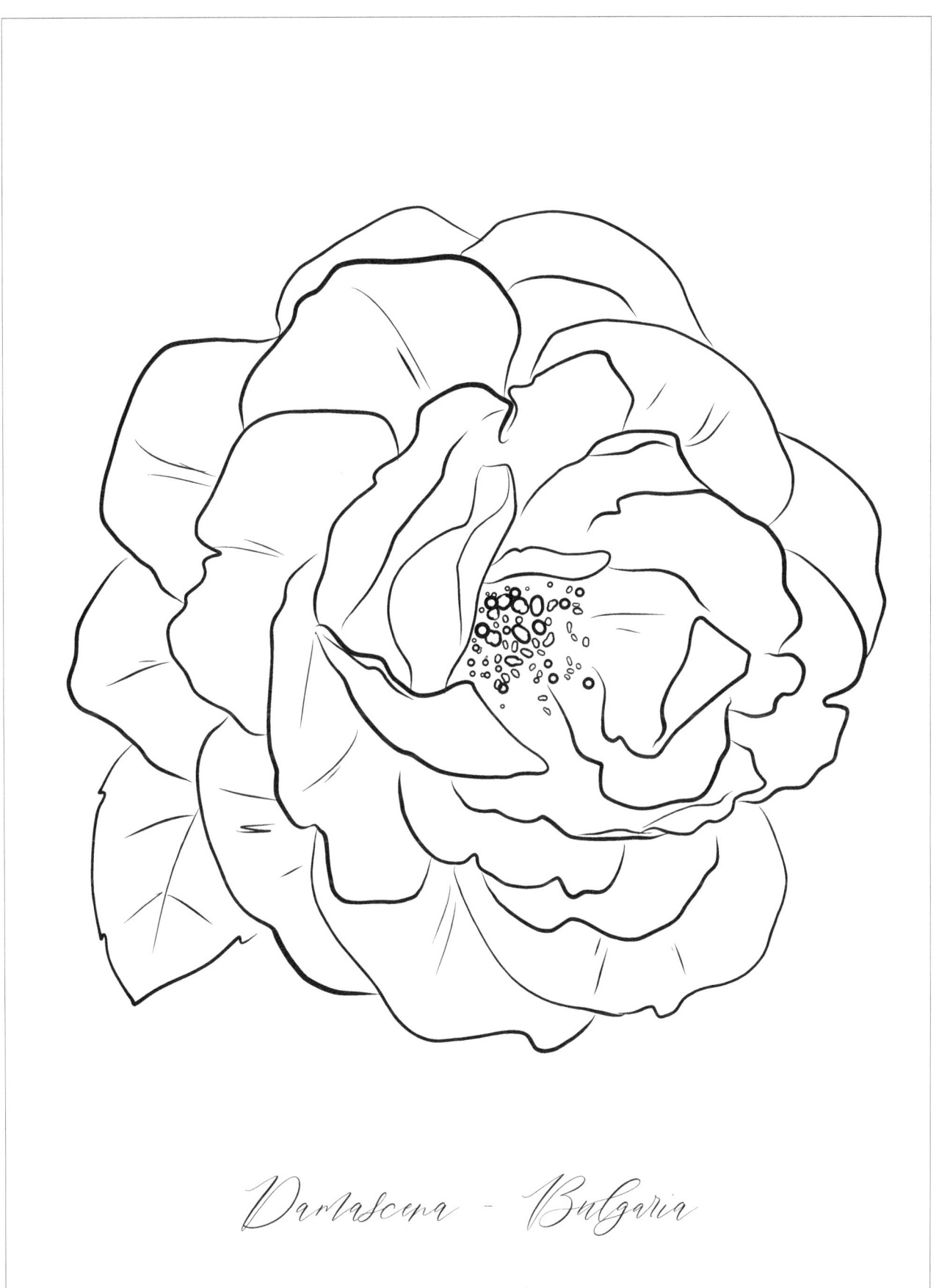

Damascena - Bulgaria

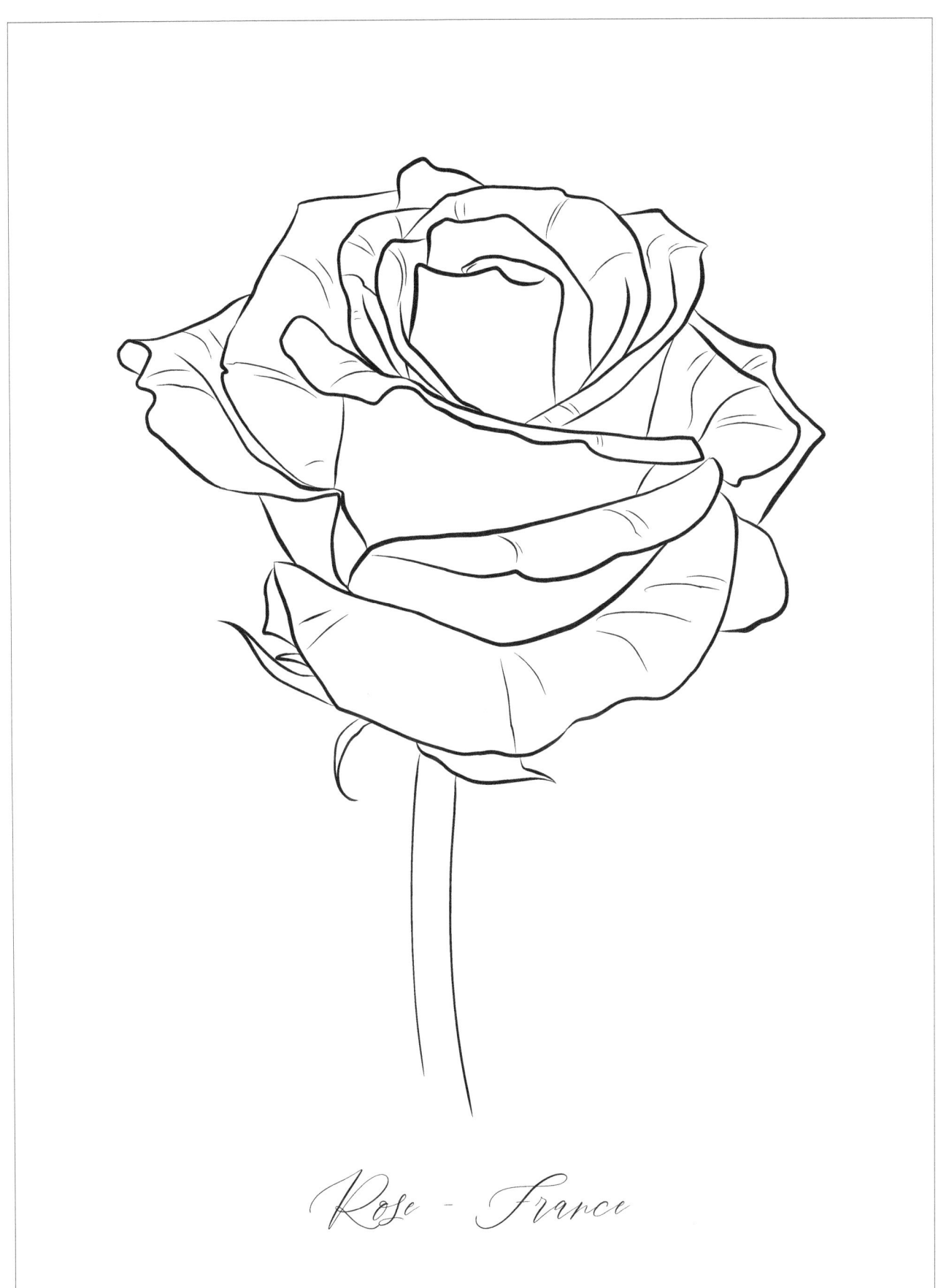

Rose - France

Scent Imagination

Look at the flower on the opposite page.
- Close your eyes
- Imagine the scent of this flower
- Imagine its color

Three Gratitude Breaths

With each of three deep breaths, silently name one thing you're grateful for. Big or small.

Affirmation Quote

My breath is my shelter. I return to it when the world feels too loud, its soothing and peaceful.

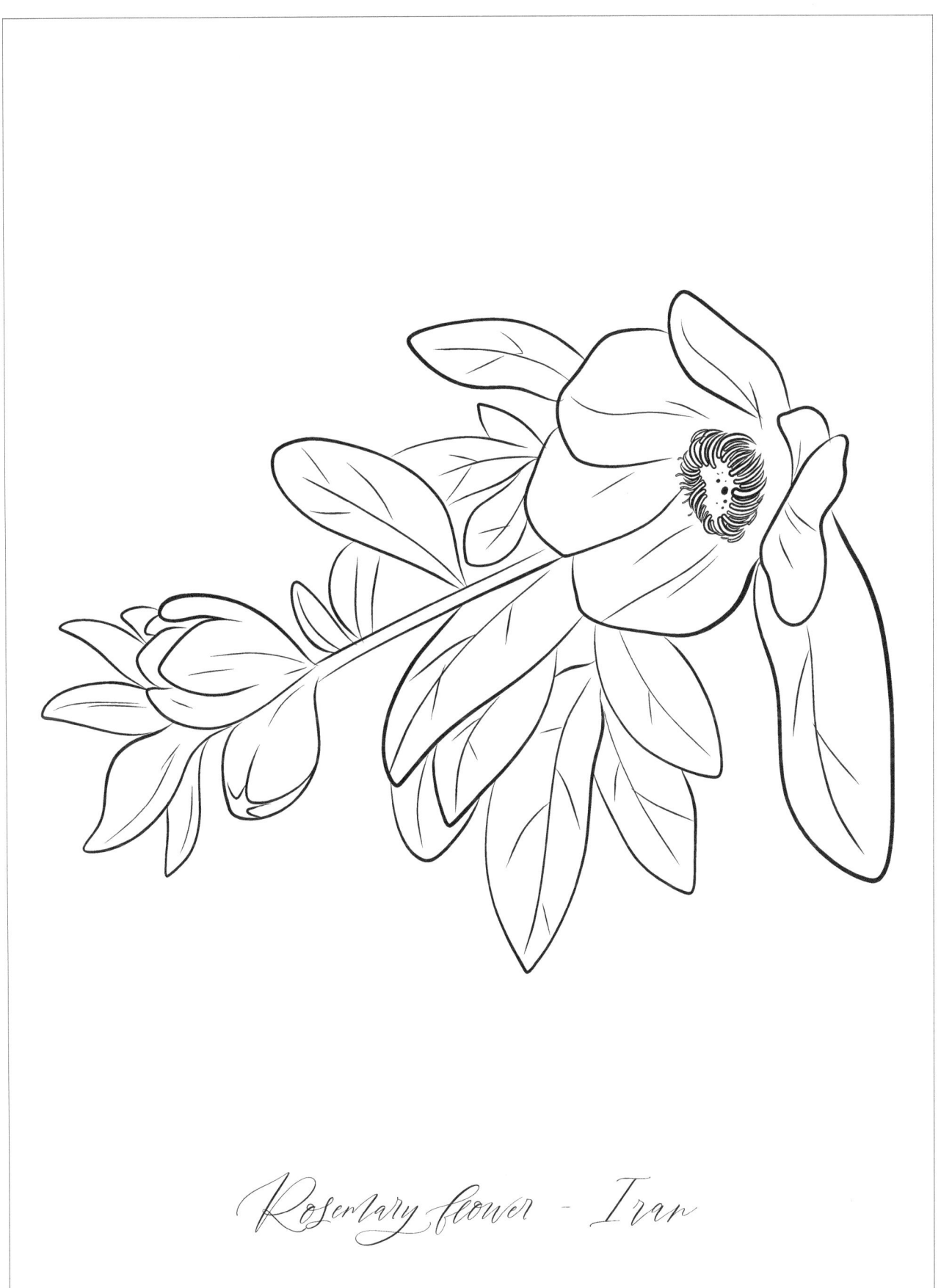

Rosemary flower - Iran

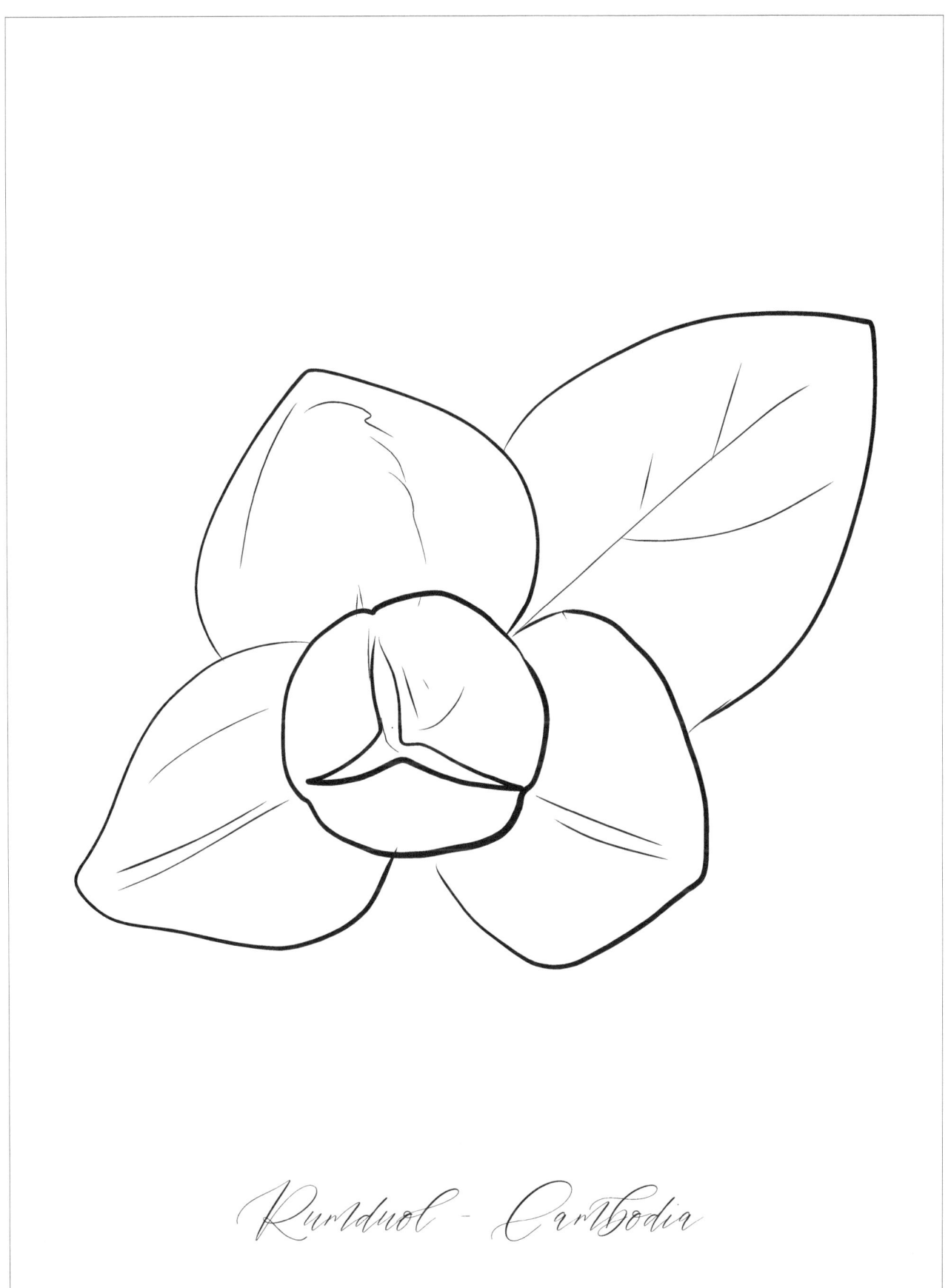

Rumduol - Cambodia

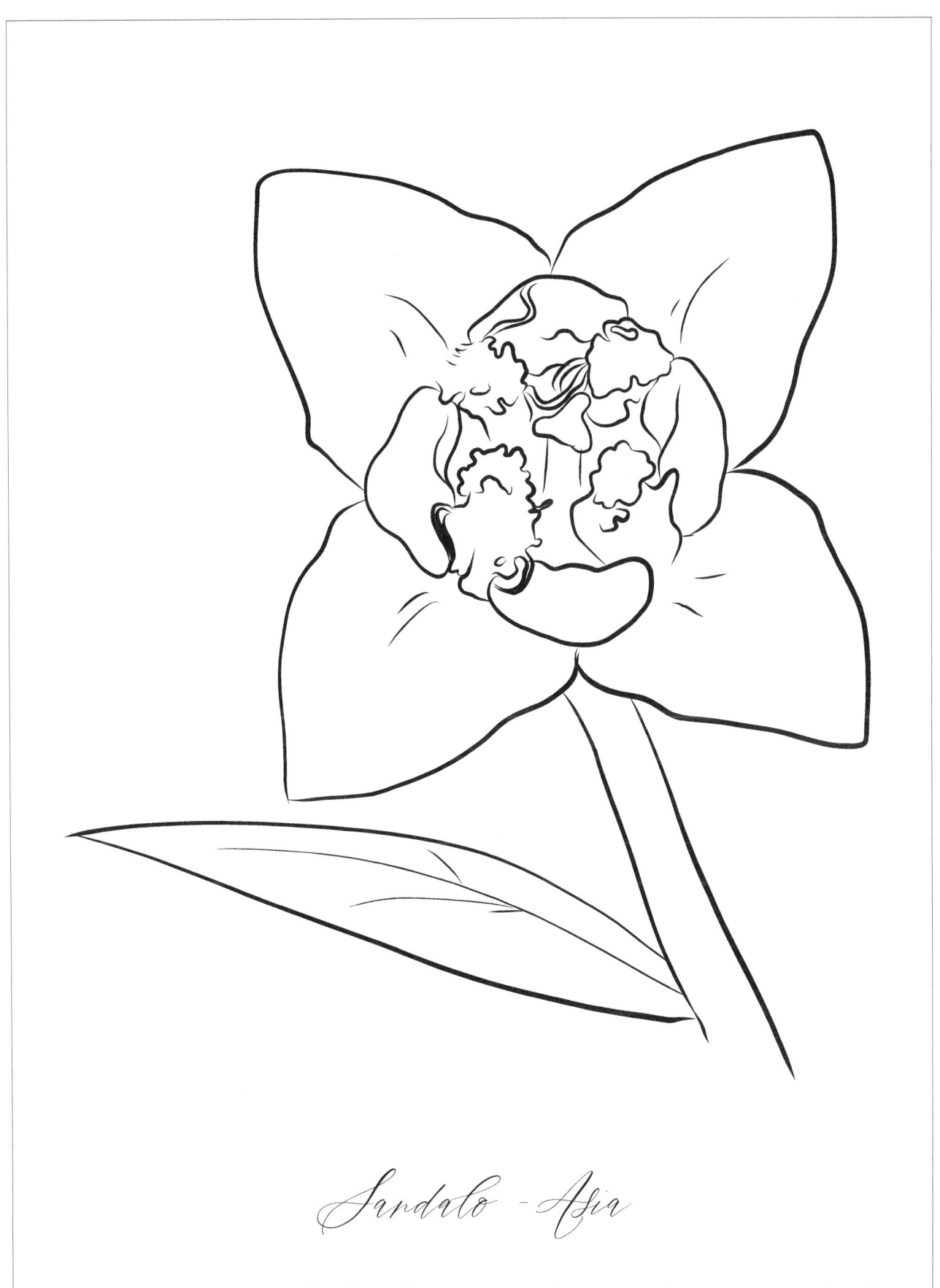

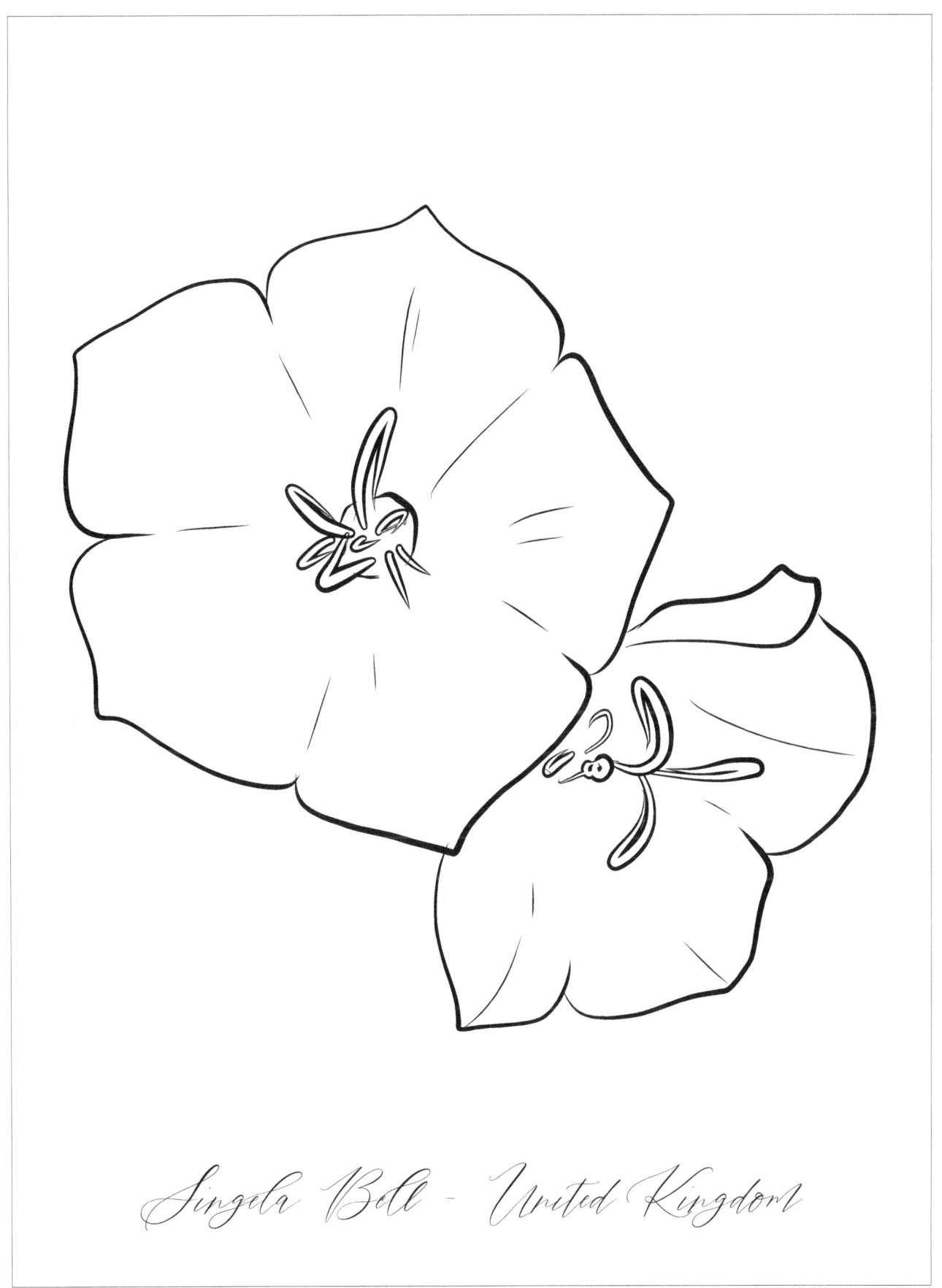

Singela Bell - United Kingdom

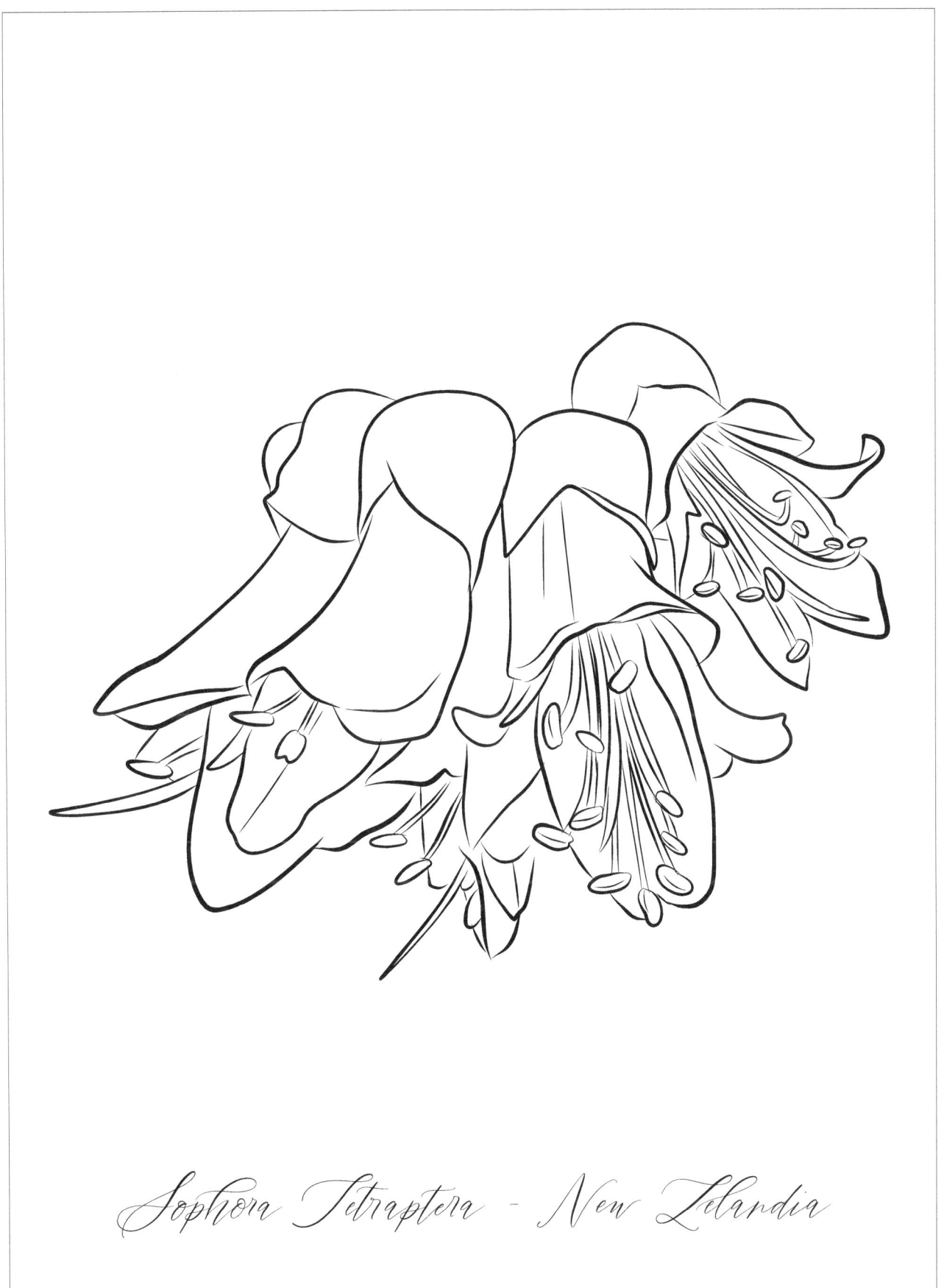

Sophora Tetraptera - New Zelandia

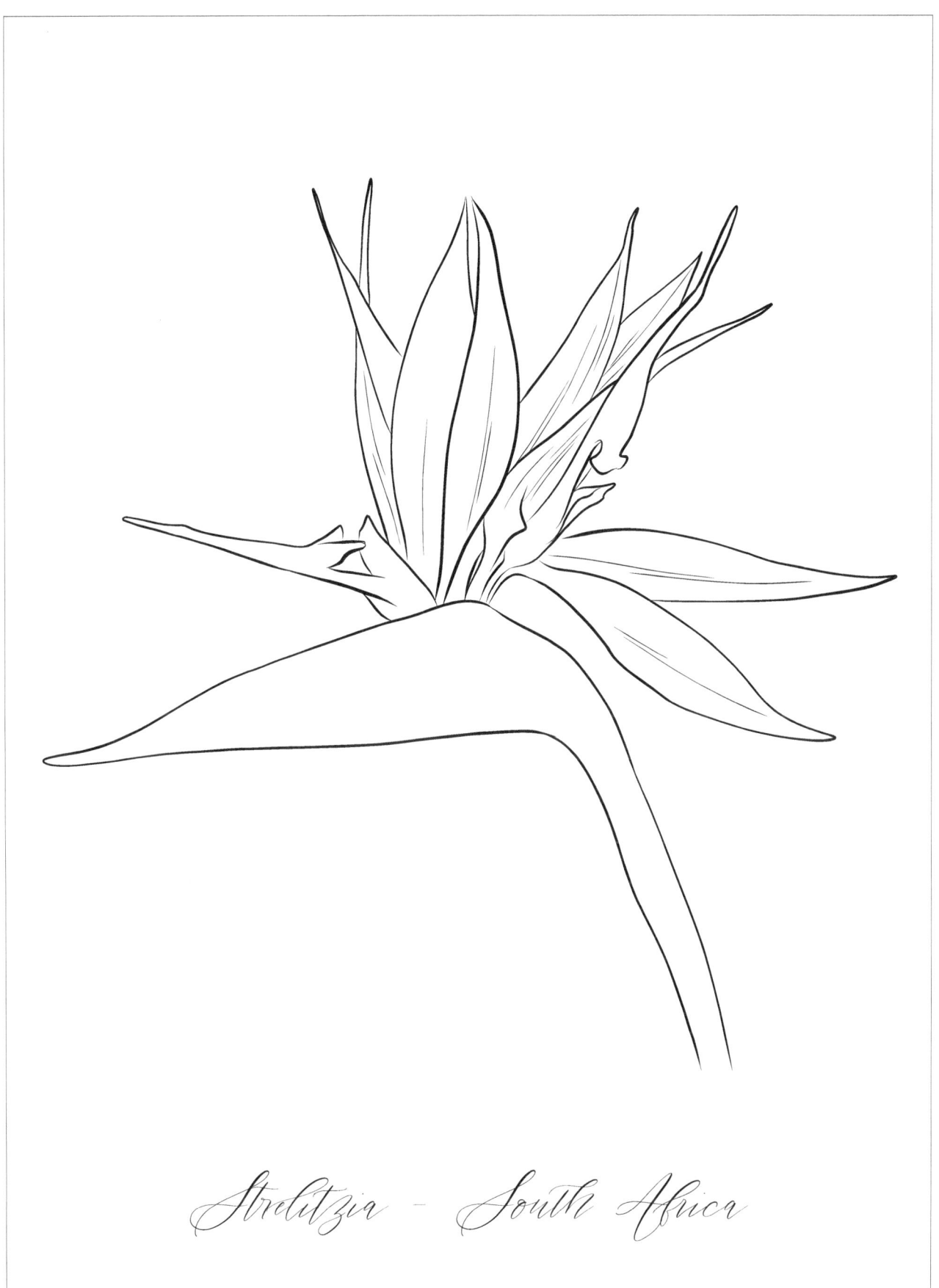

Strelitzia – South Africa

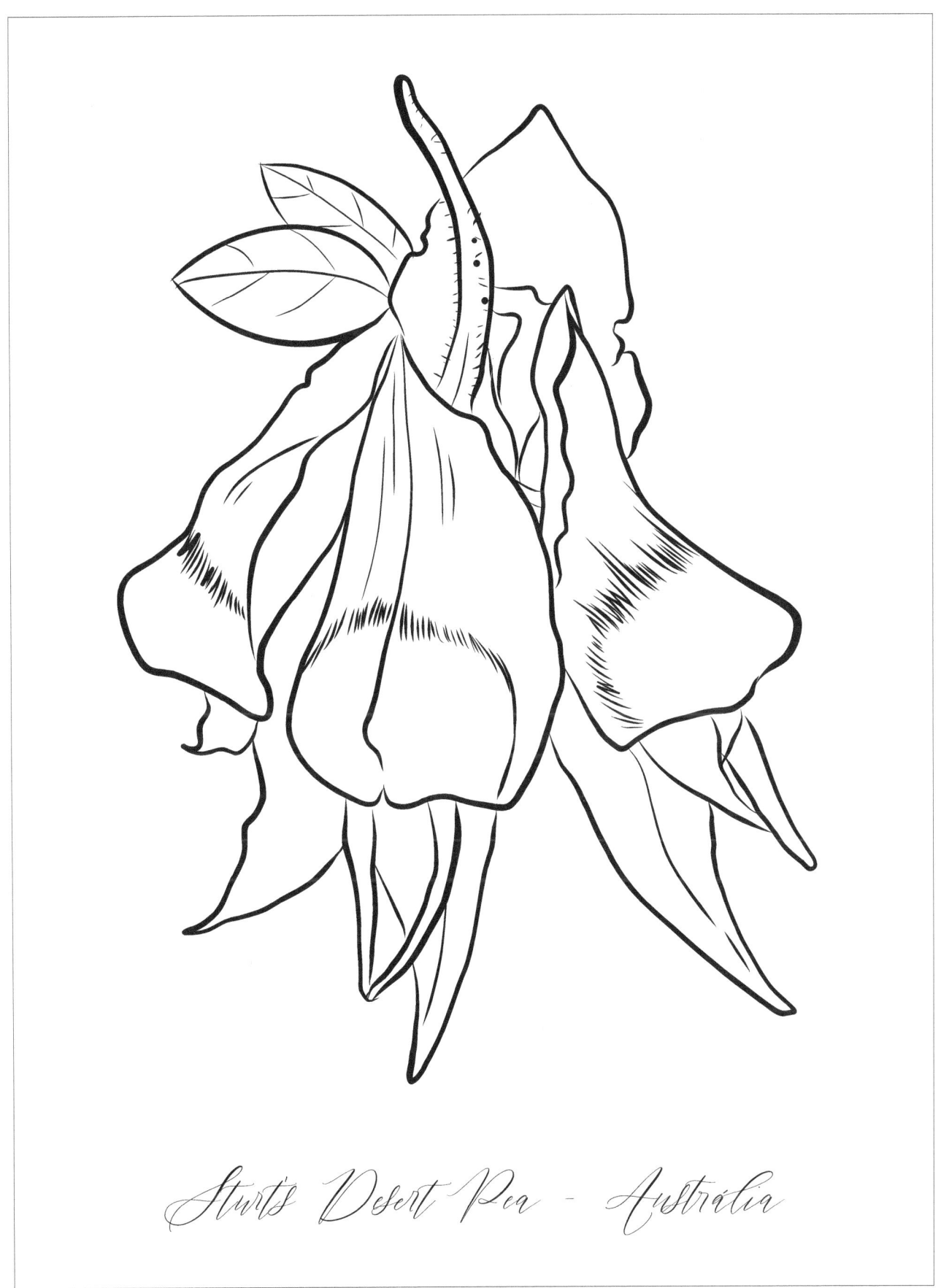

Sturt's Desert Pea - Australia

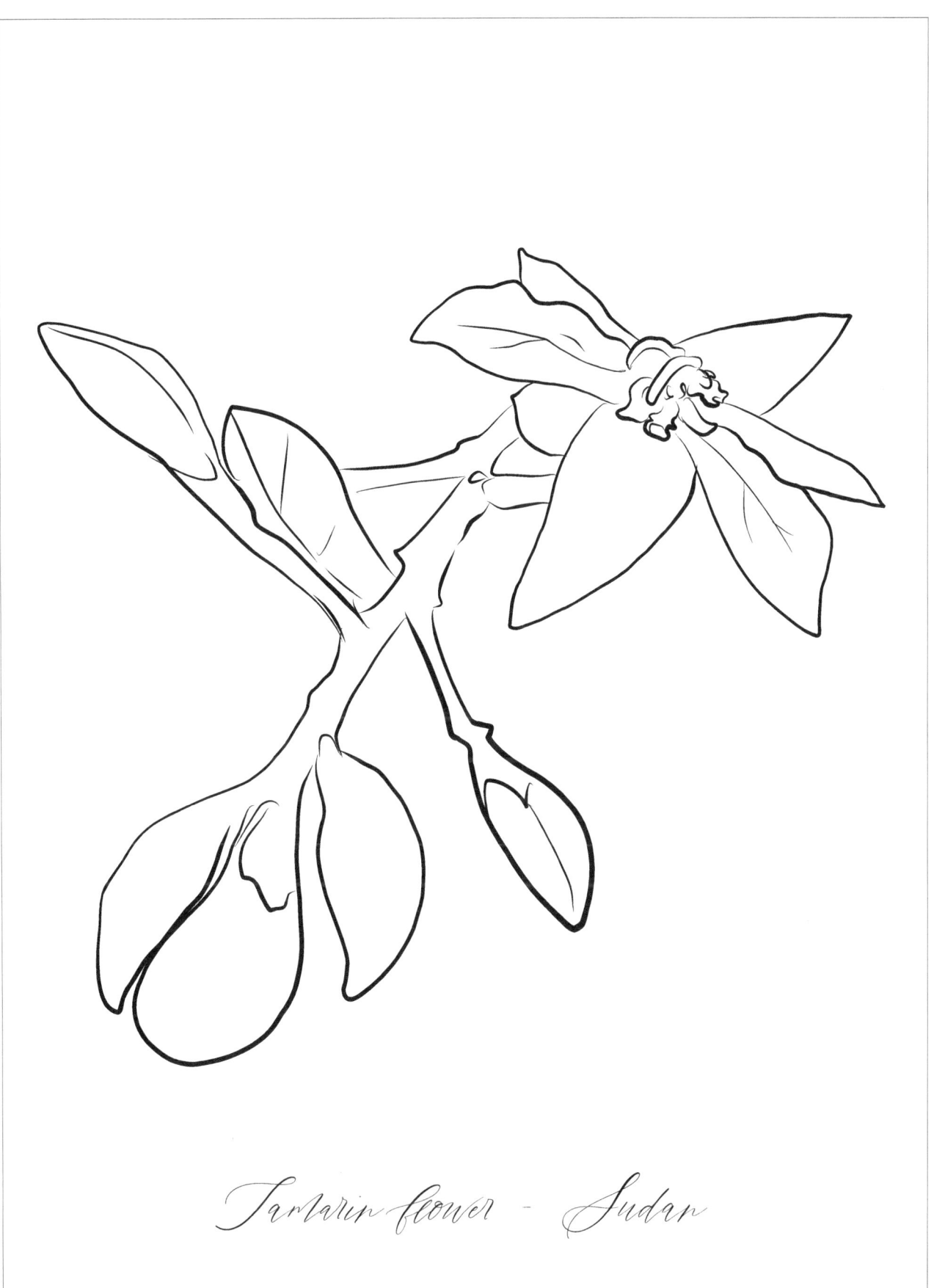

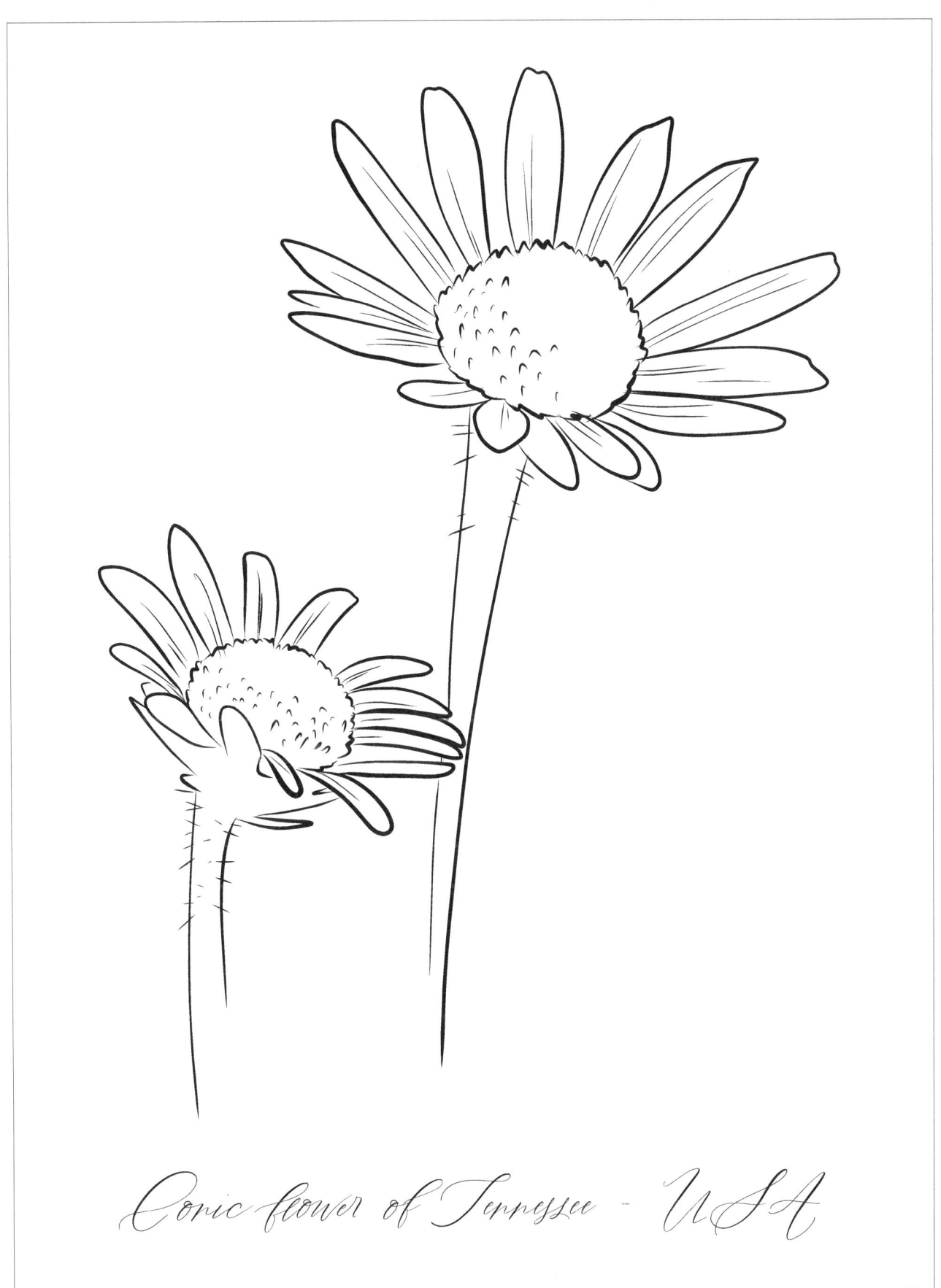

Conic flower of Tennessee - USA

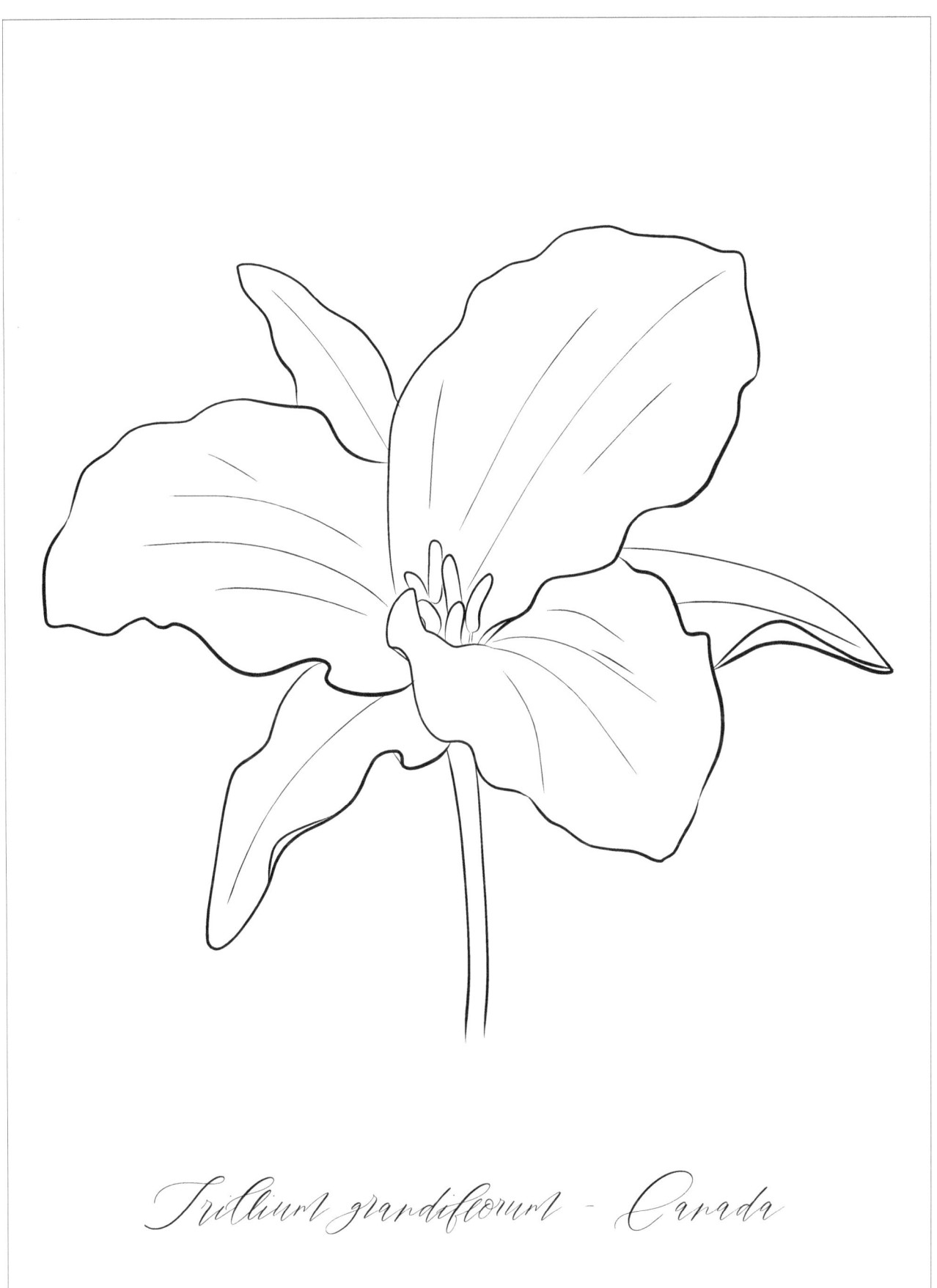

Scent Imagination

Look at the flower on the opposite page.

- Close your eyes
- Imagine the scent of this flower
- Imagine its color

Color Your Calm

Close your eyes, and as you visualize coloring, mentally say:

- *"I am here."*
- *"I am okay."*
- *"I am letting go."*

Affirmation Quote

I am safe. I am steady. I am enough, I can go on with my life to new beautiful horizons.

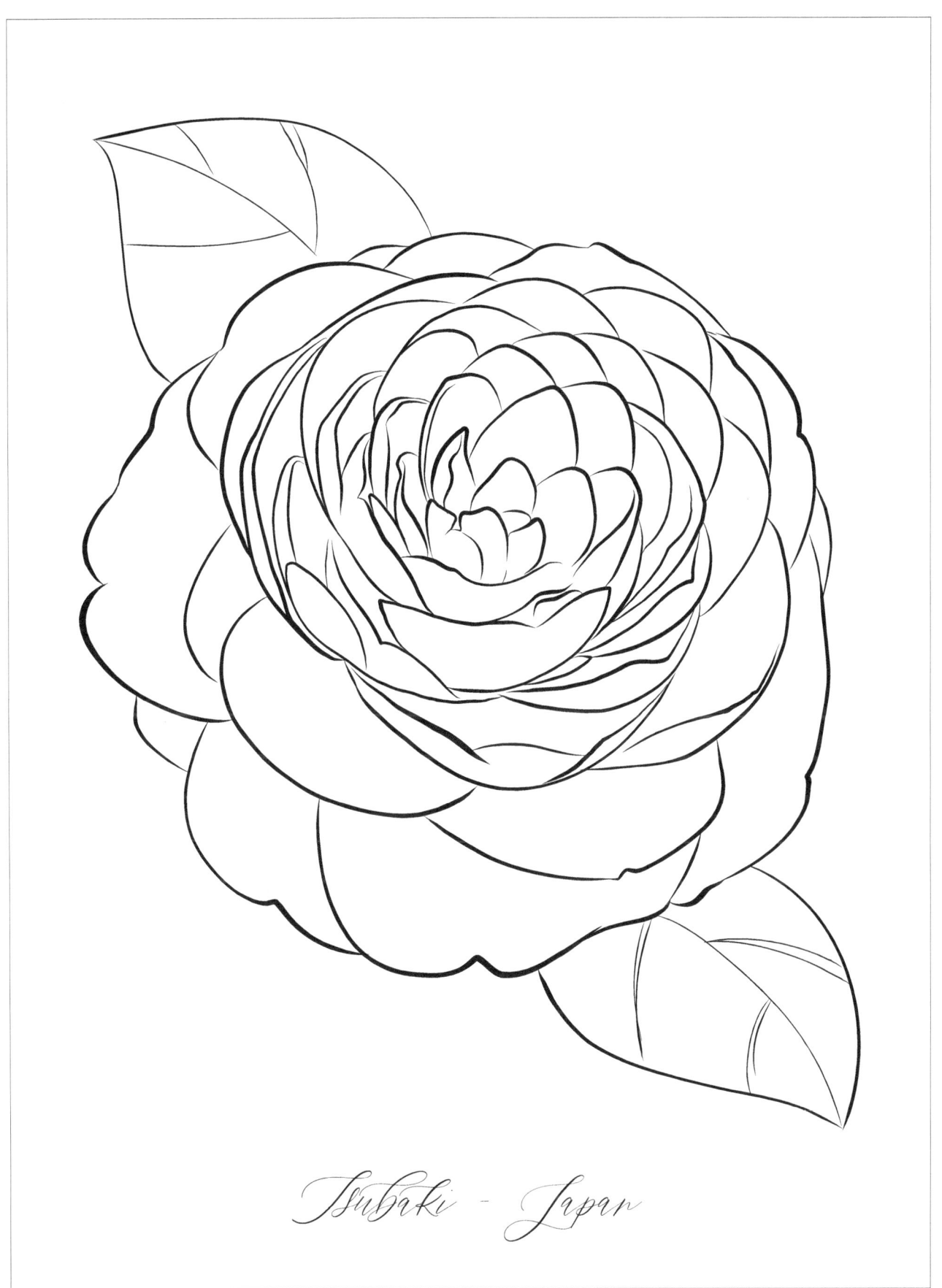

Tsubaki - Japan

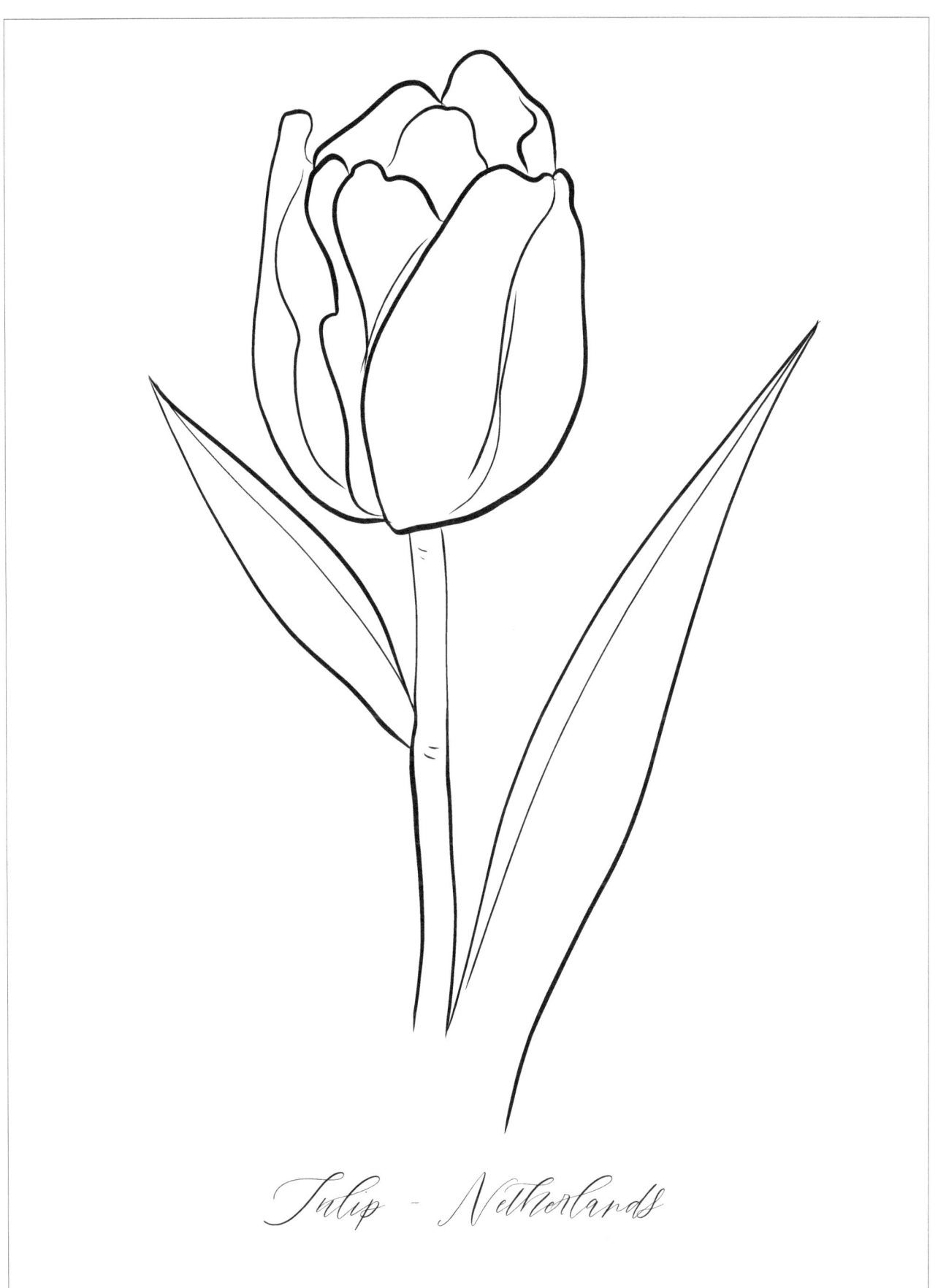

Tulip - Netherlands

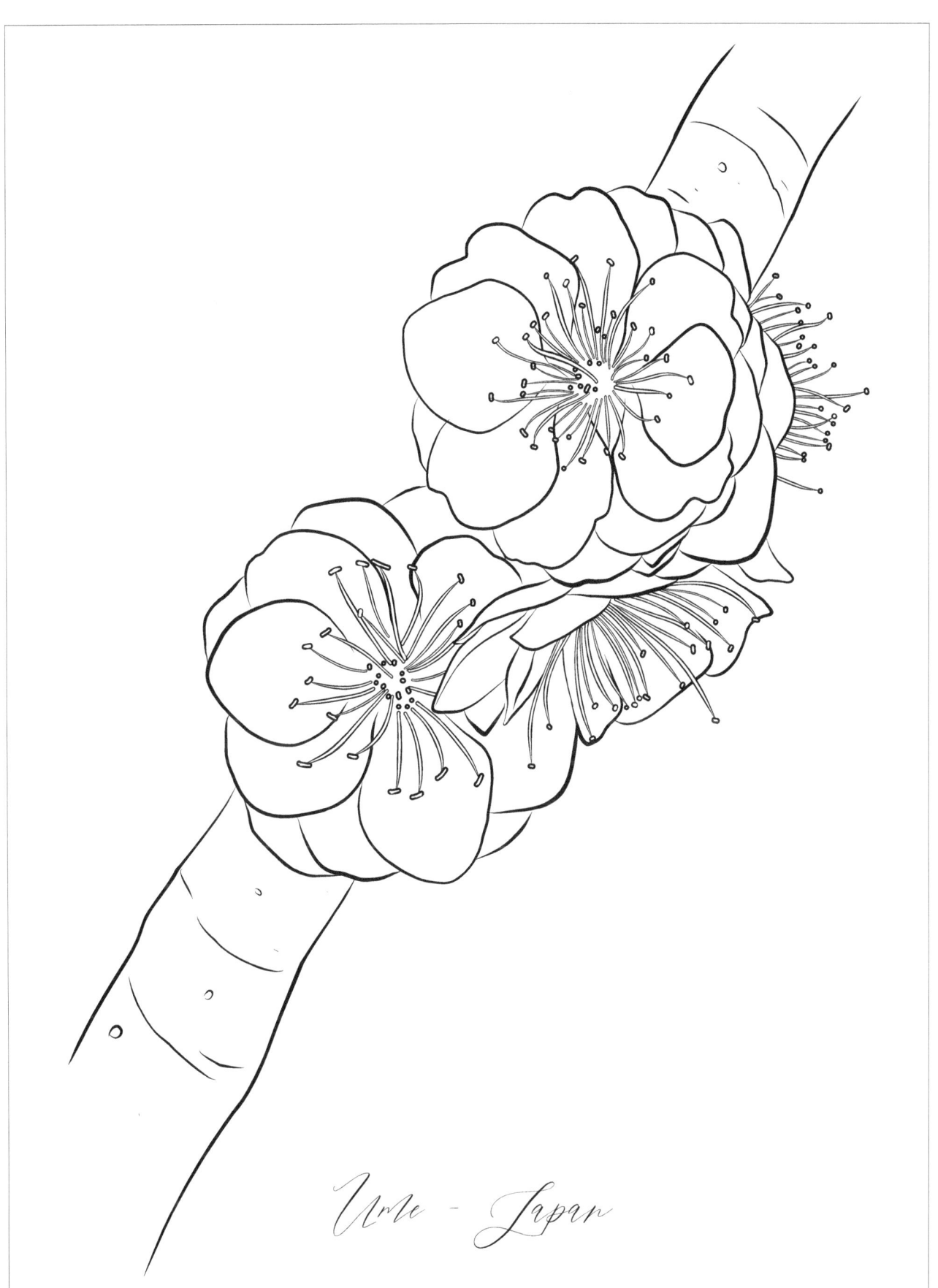

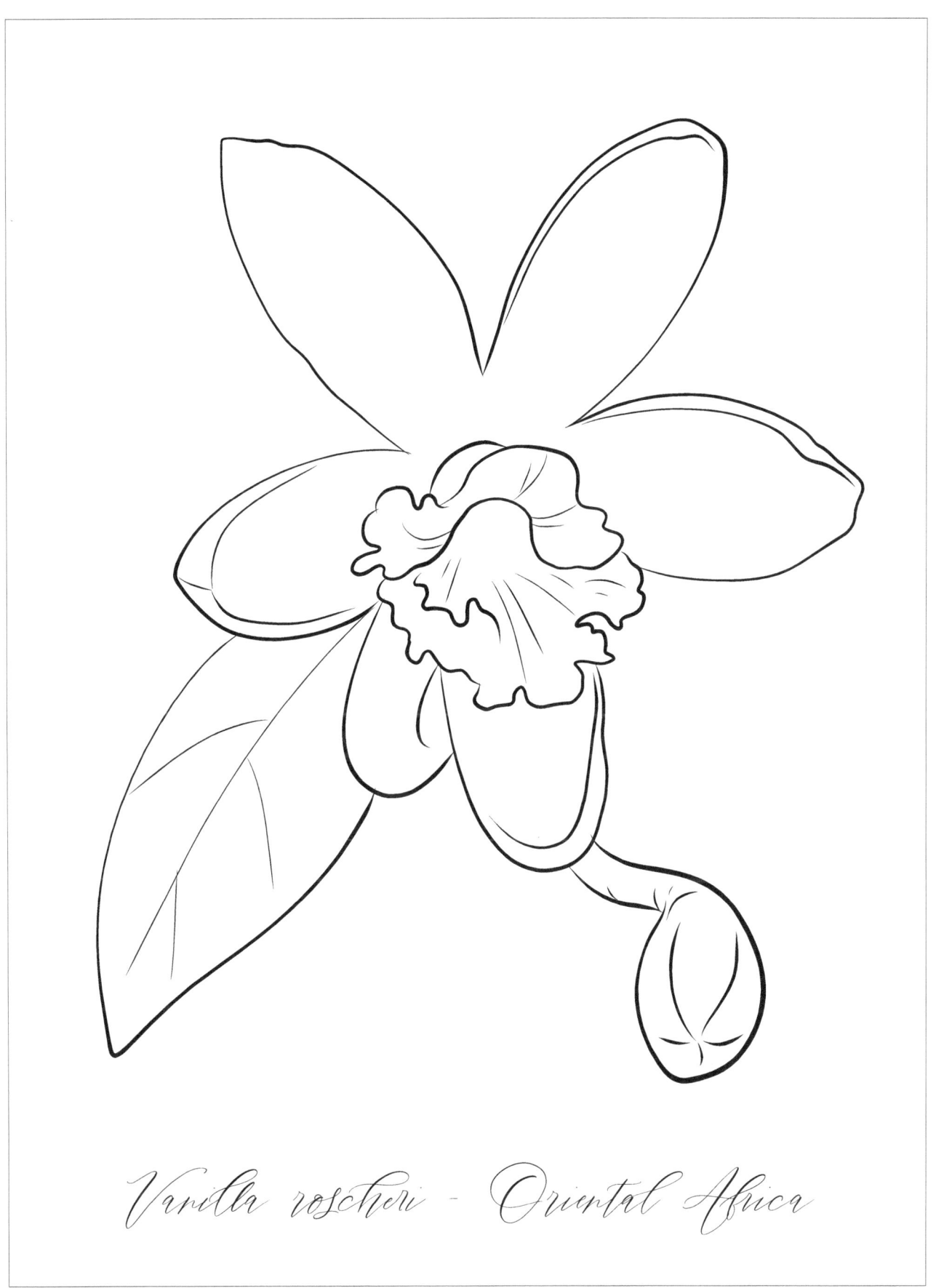

Vanilla roscheri – Oriental Africa

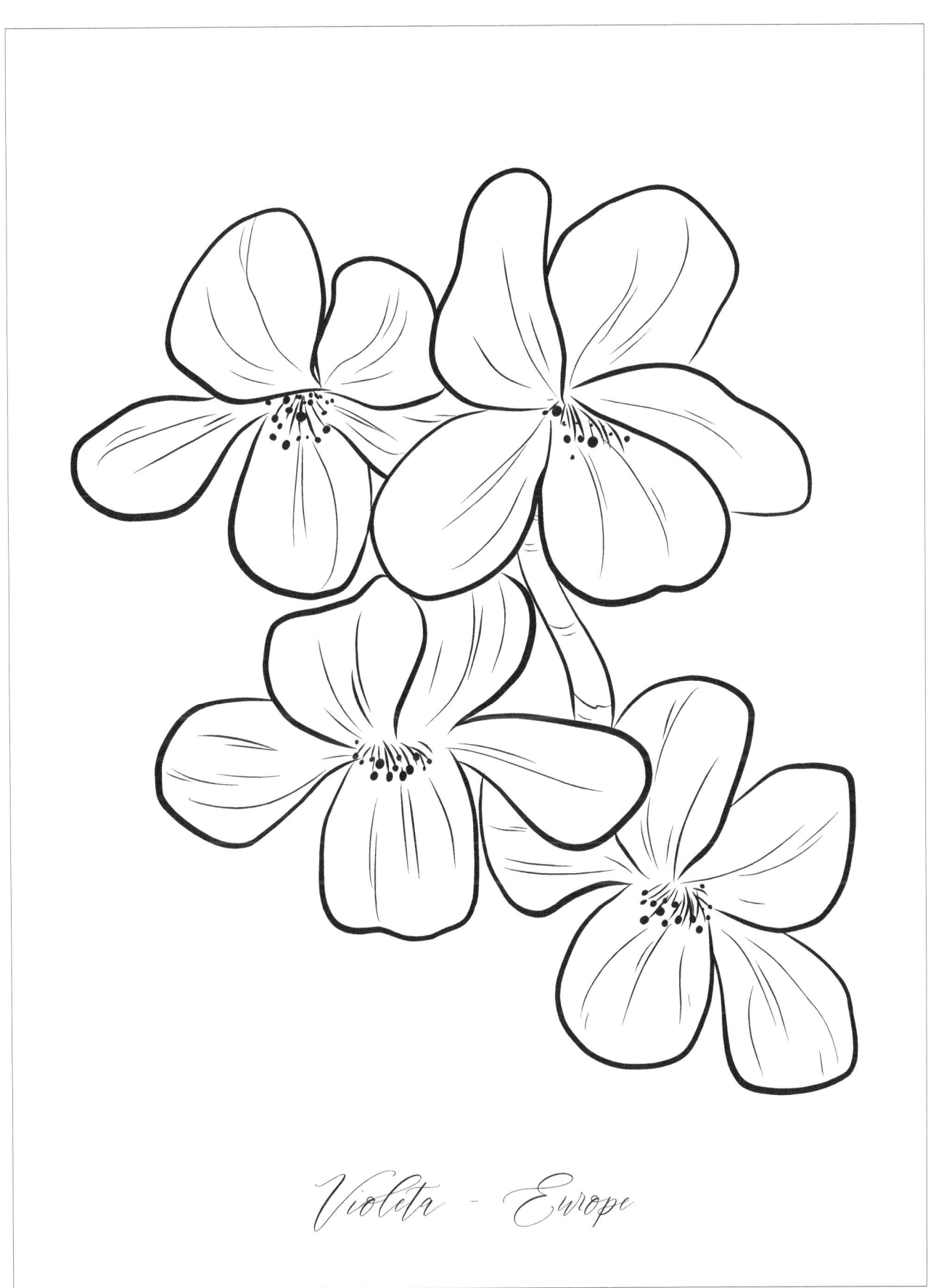

Violeta - Europe

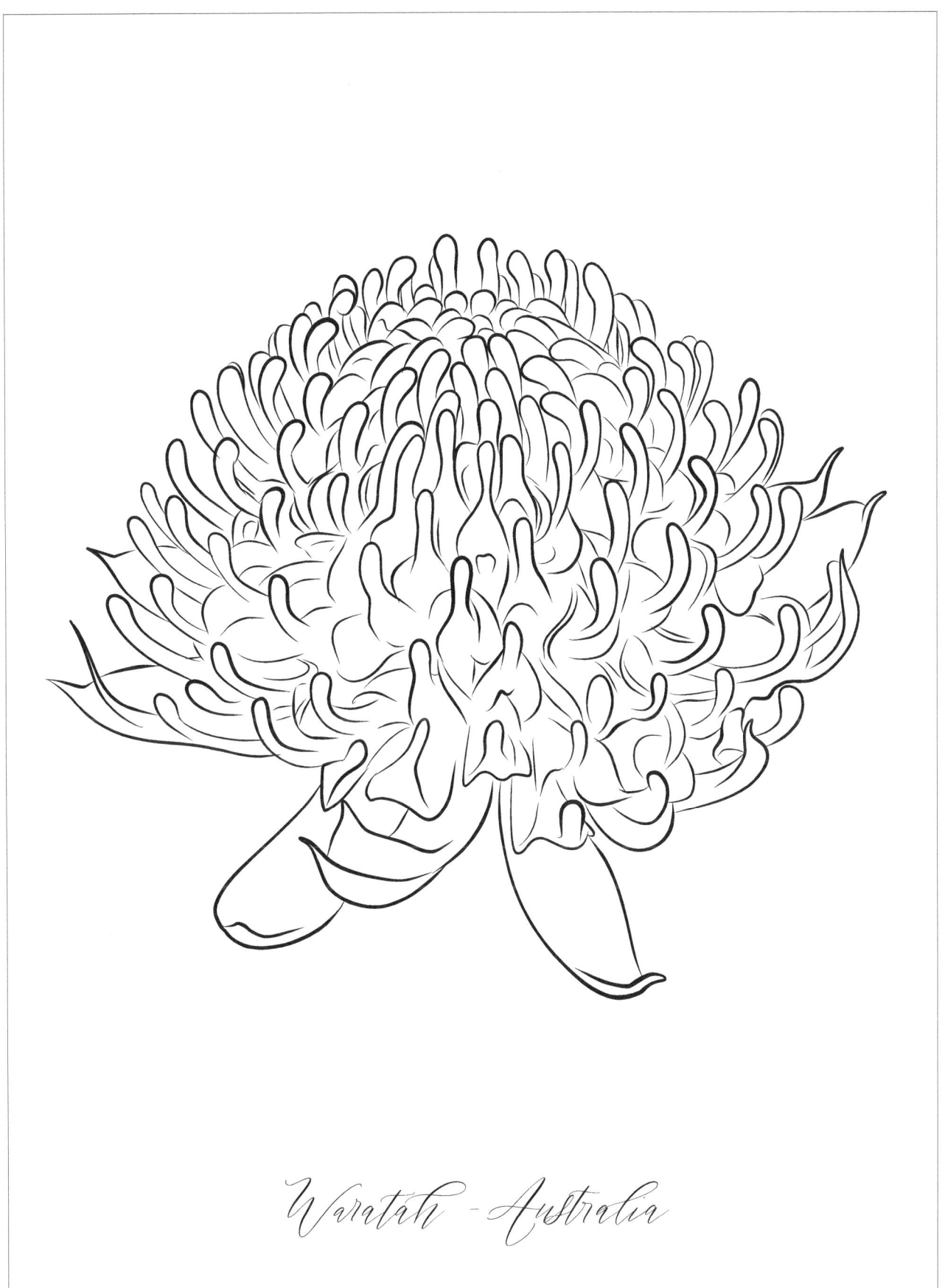

Waratah - Australia

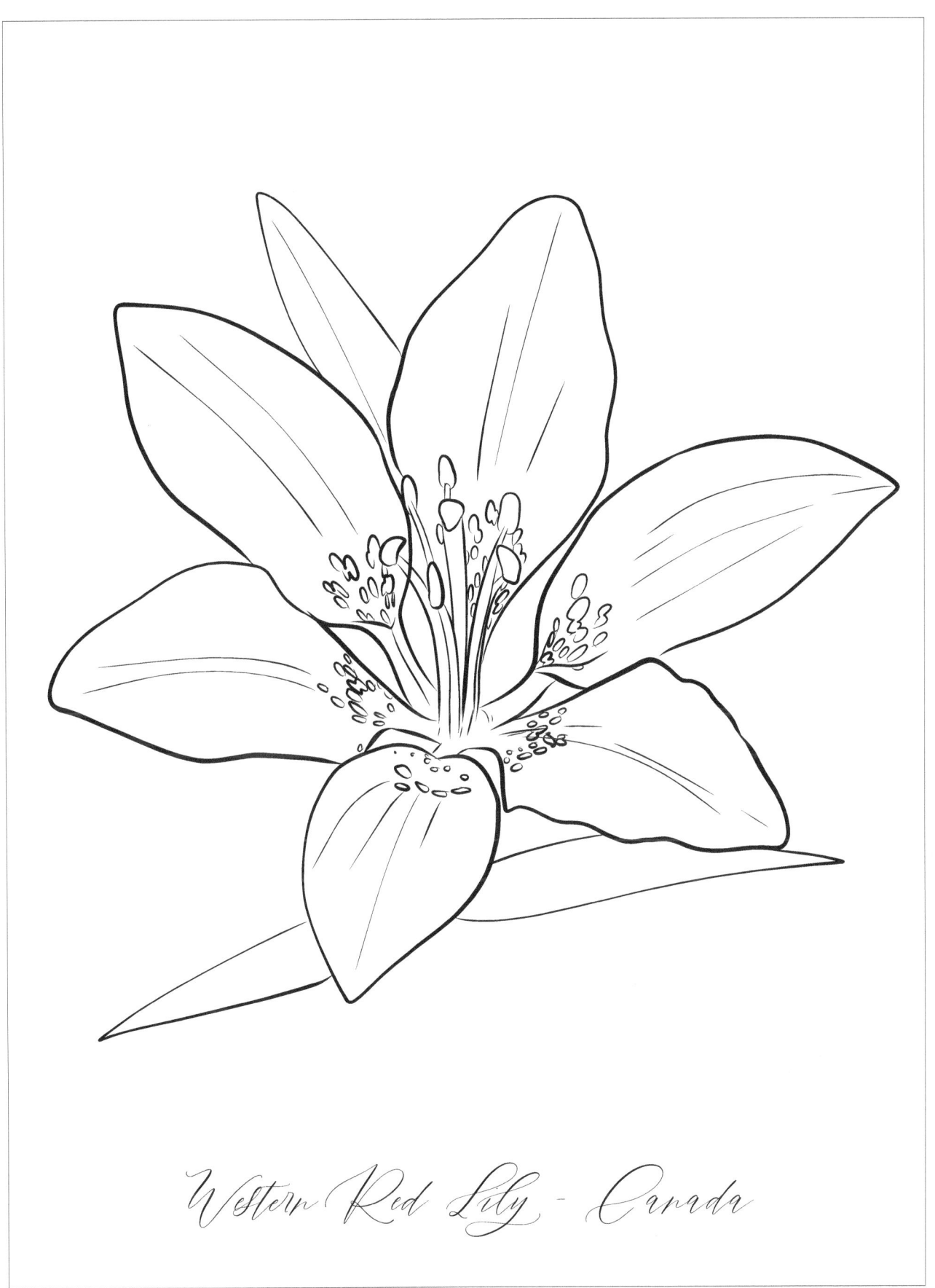

Western Red Lily - Canada

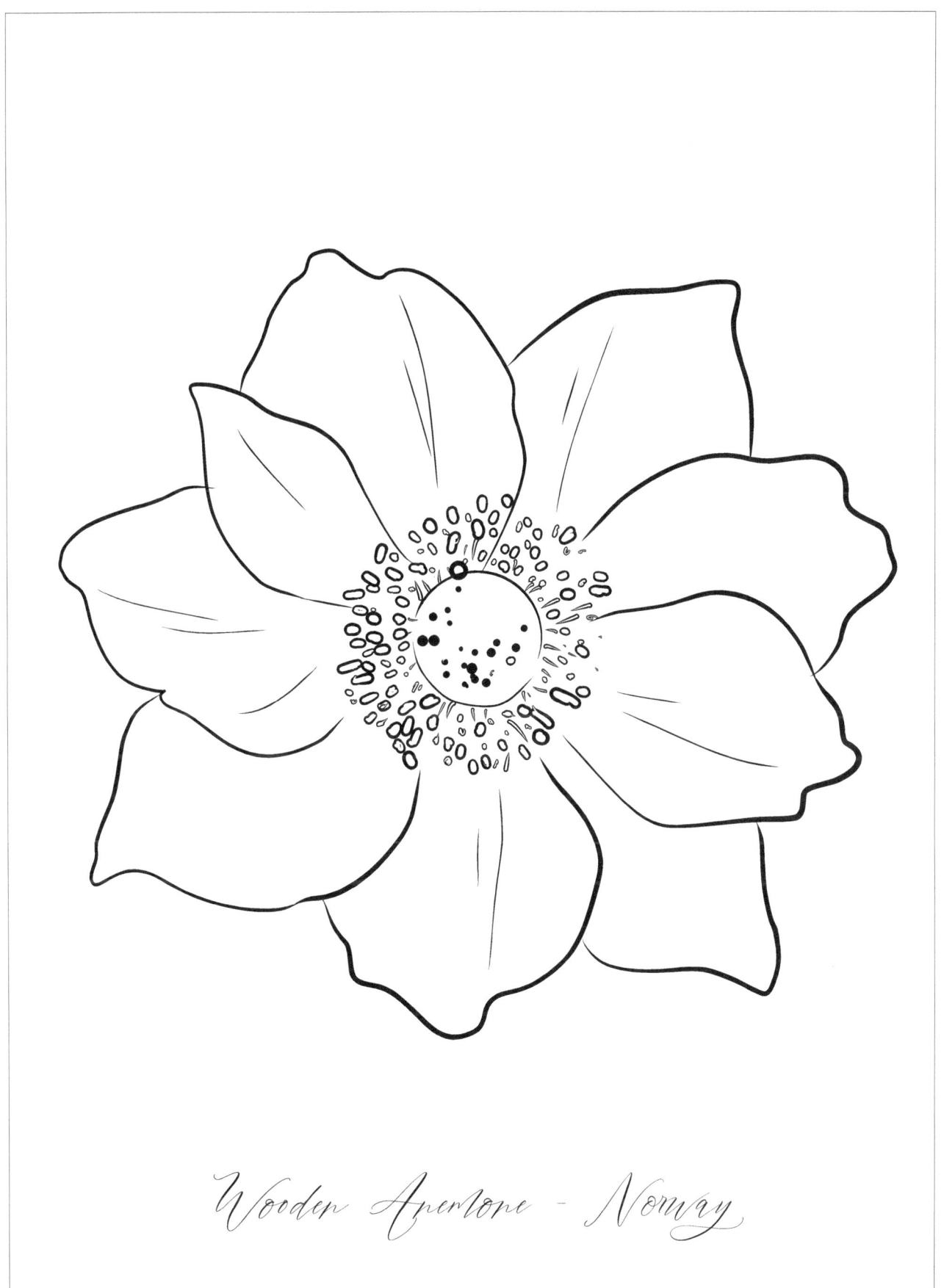

Wooden Anemone - Norway

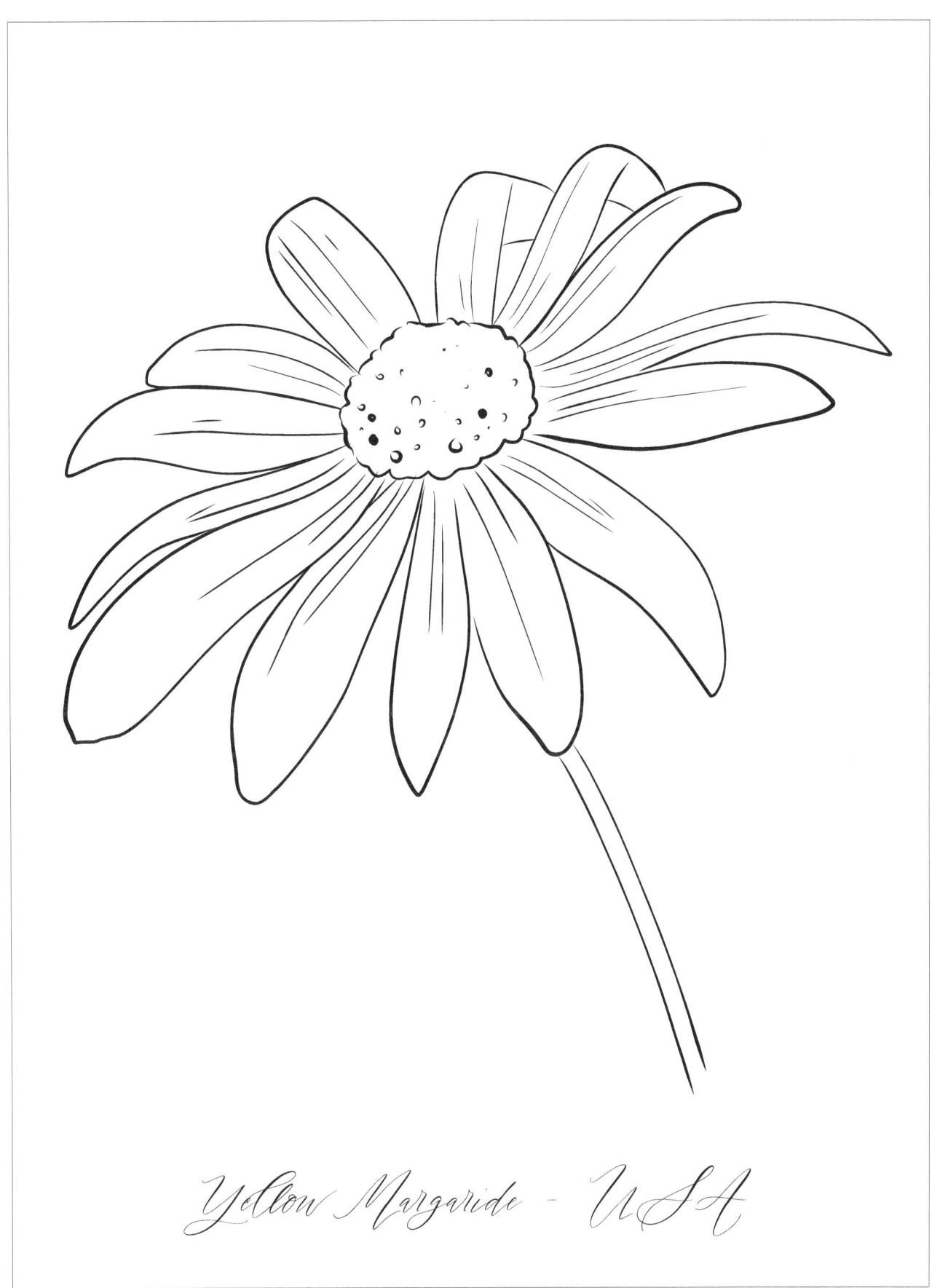

Yellow Margaride - USA

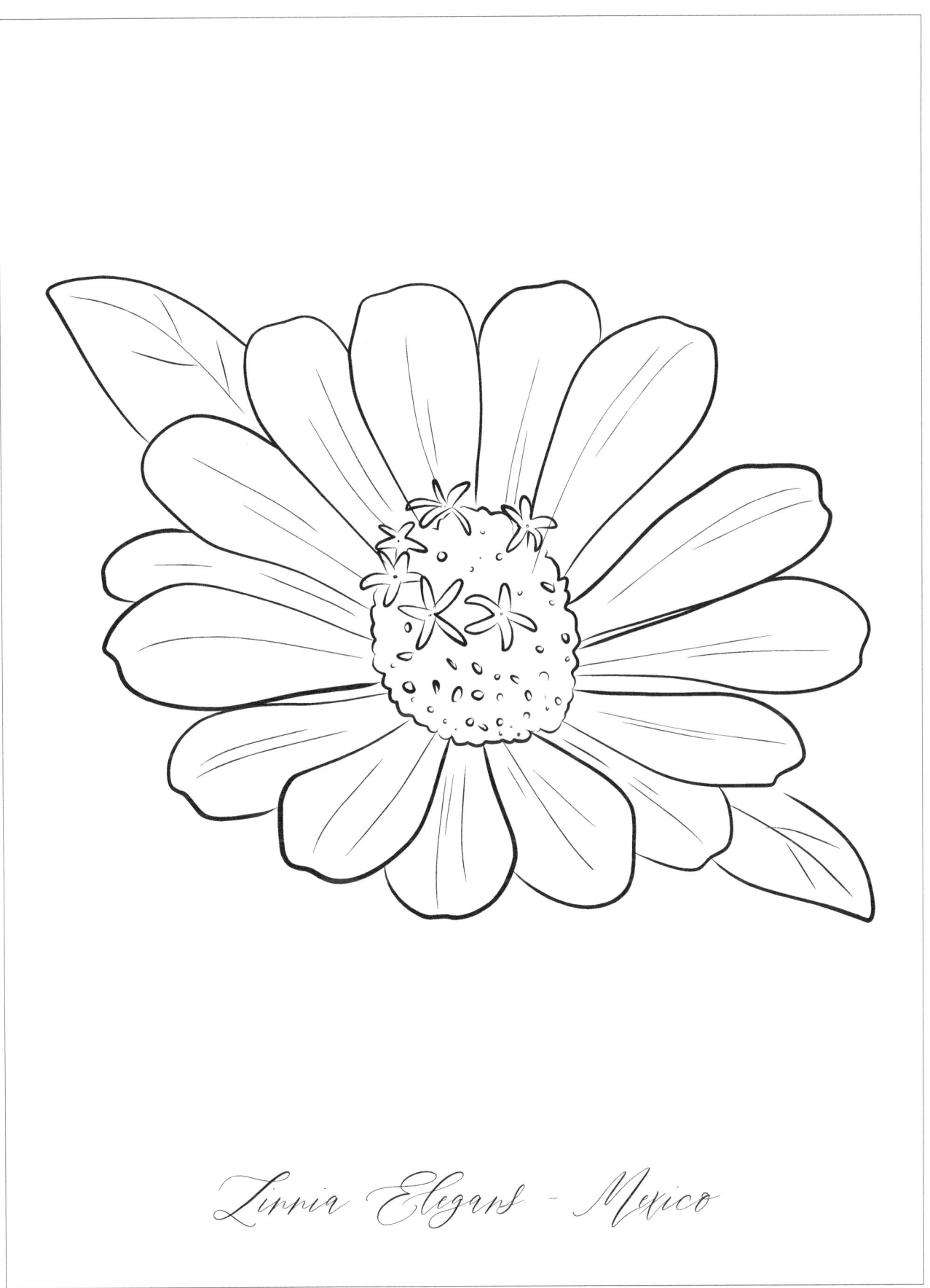

Zinnia Elegans - Mexico

Peace

www.ingramcontent.com/pod-product-compliance
Lightning Source LLC
LaVergne TN
LVHW081518060526
838200LV00006B/214